Beauty by Nature

Brigitte Mars, AHG

HEALTHY LIVING PUBLICATIONS
Summertown, Tennessee

Library of Congress Cataloging-in-Publication Data

Mars, Brigitte.
Beauty by nature / Brigitte Mars.
p. cm.
Includes bibliographical references and index.
ISBN-13: 978-1-57067-193-7 (alk. paper)
ISBN-10: 1-57067-193-1 (alk. paper)
1. Beauty, Personal. 2. Naturopathy. 3. Health. I. Title.

RA776.98.M375 2006
646.7'042—dc22 2006025181

DISCLAIMER

Beauty by Nature was written to help you take more responsibility for your own health and beauty. Should you find that any natural remedies are not working for you, or if you have a negative reaction to them, please consult with a competent health professional. But remember, *you* should be your primary health care provider!

15 14 13 12 11 10 09 08 07 06 1 2 3 4 5 6 7 8 9

Cover and Interior design: Aerocraft Charter Art Service
Cover photos: (upper left) Mickel Roberts, makeup by Hope Zarro
(lower left) Rainbeau Mars, life guide
(center) Plush Studios (Adobe)
(lower right) Adobe
Back cover photo: © 2006 Jeff Boxer
Interior photos: page 91, 92 Guy Ziau
pages 158–161 © 2006 Jeff Boxer
Illustrations: page 133, Swan Palermo

Printed in Canada

Healthy Living Publications
A division of Book Publishing Company
P.O. Box 99
Summertown, TN 38483
888-260-8458

ISBN-13: 978-1-57067-193-7
ISBN-10: 1-57067-193-1

Printed on recycled paper

The Book Publishing Co. is committed to preserving ancient forests and natural resources. We have elected to print this title at Transcontinental Printing on Enviro Antique Natural, which is 100% postconsumer recycled and processed chlorine free. As a result of our paper choice, we have saved the following natural resources:

82 trees
3,820 lbs of solid waste
29,751 gallons of water
7,167 lbs pounds of greenhouse gases
57 million BTUs of total energy
(Calculations from www.papercalculator.org)

We are a member of Green Press Initiative. For more information about Green Press Initiative visit: www.greenpressinitiative.org

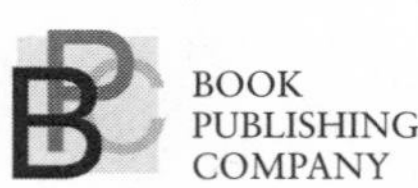

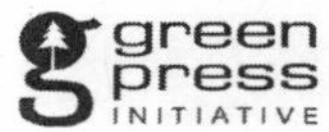

DEDICATION

This book is dedicated to my beautiful and amazing daughters,
Sunflower Sparkle Mars and Rainbeau Harmony Mars,
and my precious grandchildren,
Chiara Jade Destiny Mars and Solwyn Forest Mars Stegall.
May you walk in beauty always!

Tom Pfeiffer, you are forever my hero.

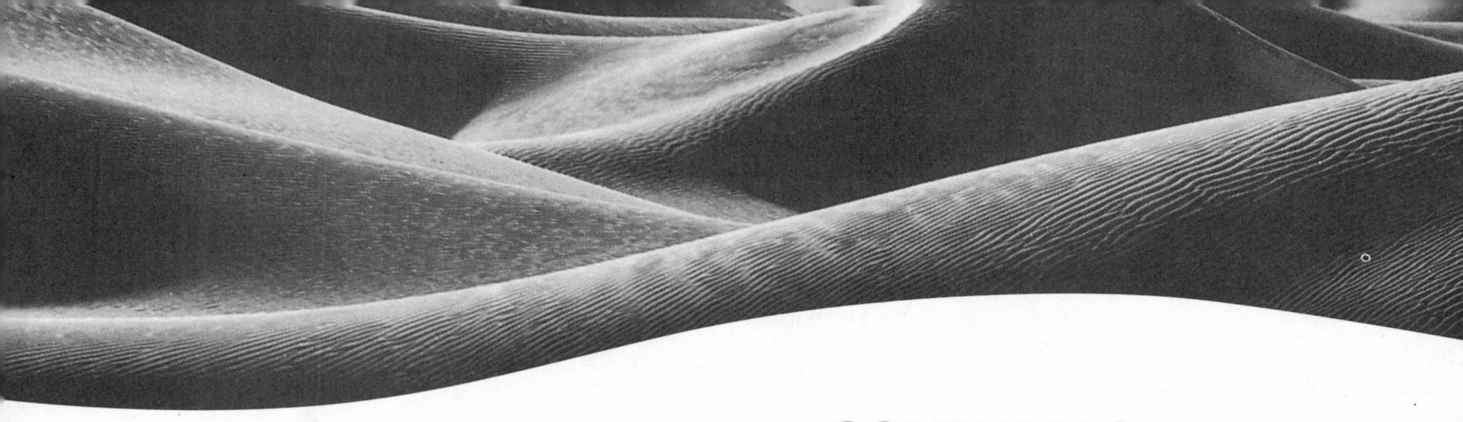

CONTENTS

FOREWORD

Ever Fortunate Reader,

You've just opened the pages to a wonderful gift. It's no coincidence that you've been guided to this book *in the present moment* . . . and here we are. This is precisely the place where we change *anything* and *everything* in our lives—how we think, how we feel, what we attract, and much more. Specifically, this book is about shifting and transforming how you perceive "beauty," giving you access to an abundance of proven beauty secrets—secrets the mainstream works so hard to suppress. Each principle you uncover will shine like the brilliant radiance of the sun, helping illuminate each step of this life-changing journey. I urge you to use the infinite power of this present moment to take full advantage of the amazing secrets you're about to discover.

To me, a person is "beautiful" to the extent that he or she is *fully immersed in wholeness*. In order to arrive at genuine "wholeness" we must let go of the things that we are not. Things that take us away from our essence divide us inside. Unfortunately, so many myths have been perpetuated about beauty that it is all too easy to get caught in the trap of believing them. We are all familiar with many common, unwholesome approaches—pharmaceutical drugs, chemical-based products, maybe even surgery. Of course, what has been our "past" does not have to be our future. And that's why you hold such a treasure in your hands!

You see, my mother has a million and one ways to nurture your *real beauty*, each incredible tip assisting you in this wonderful return to wholeness. I humbly ask that you stay open to each piece of guidance and allow yourself to be taken back to the true source of beauty that exists inside us all.

I did not realize the series of incredible gifts I had access to while growing up. Now I can gratefully say that so much of what I do and give to the world is a reflection of what I learned from my mother. Much like my mother's work, my own job is to illuminate and guide others on the path to self-love and beauty. Some of the most successful and "beautiful" people from around the world have sought my assistance in this area, and I never could have come to this point without the privilege of absorbing my mother's wisdom. I thank my mom immensely for taking the time to write this book. There's never been a better time or more need for such a powerful message. I know her knowledge comes from a very deep place in her heart, a place of true service and contribution.

Nearly every one of these powerful principles contained in *Beauty by Nature* has been around for thousands of years. They are backed by more evidence of success than any chemical or surgical procedure. I pray that enlightened individuals like you will carry the torch, sharing them with future generations.

In this book, you will find the natural health and beauty wisdom of countless generations. Each principle was trusted and brought down through the ages and has been tested by millions of beautiful, aware individuals . . . just like yourself. With no chemicals and nothing artificial to manufacture, our ancestors relied solely upon nature to nurture and perfect their bodies. Nature has and always will hold the answers to deep and radiant beauty, if we remain open to it. The more we understand this, the more absurd it seems that someone would trust a bright fluorescent-colored potion that has not a single ingredient that the average person can even pronounce! Yet we're told that if we scrub our faces with it, it will make us beautiful.

If the creator (and the source of all things) has anything to offer us in the way of real beauty, you will find it in this book. This book is for those who truly intend to unveil the full potential of their beauty, who seek expert guidance on this magical path. This book will enlighten you on how to use food and herbs to enhance your skin, nails, hair, and figure—anything and everything that could make you look and feel more beautiful *naturally.* Most importantly, as you reconnect with your source, you'll begin to naturally glow and emanate beauty like never before. I know because I've seen it happen in myself, in countless numbers of both everyday people and celebrity clients, and most especially in my mother herself. She honestly looks younger and more vibrant with each passing year.

I would also like to add that the information revealed in the following pages is not only practical, it's fun! What woman wouldn't want to take nightly, luxurious baths using exotic essential oils or enjoy a foot massage to stimulate the sensual nerves in her feet and all the organs of her body? I can't imagine not being able to soothe my face with an exotic mask, feeling that I've just wonderfully nurtured not only my skin but my inner love and acceptance. I'm always amazed at how my mother has pored through thousands of books and magazines about beauty, even those that would seem utterly whimsical to the average health expert. And how she's developed such a world-class knack for extracting the most useful and pleasurable secrets of health and beauty, instantly communicating them in a simple, immediately accessible way.

I believe you've been drawn to this book because you desire something deeper—an element of beauty that intuitively you feel exists yet remains hidden from the public eye. If so, you've come to the right place. This is the most comprehensive and easy-to-use manual for acquiring, feeling, and radiating *beauty* on all levels of your being. If you take the advice that follows to heart, I promise your life will be changed forever.

How do I know? Because it has changed my life and the life of every single person I've ever shared this information with. Just read, keep your mind and heart open, put the advice into practice, and beauty beyond your wildest dreams will emerge. It is your birthright.

In love and true beauty,

Rainbeau Mars
www.rainbeaumars.com
Artist for *Yoga for Beauty* videos and DVDs

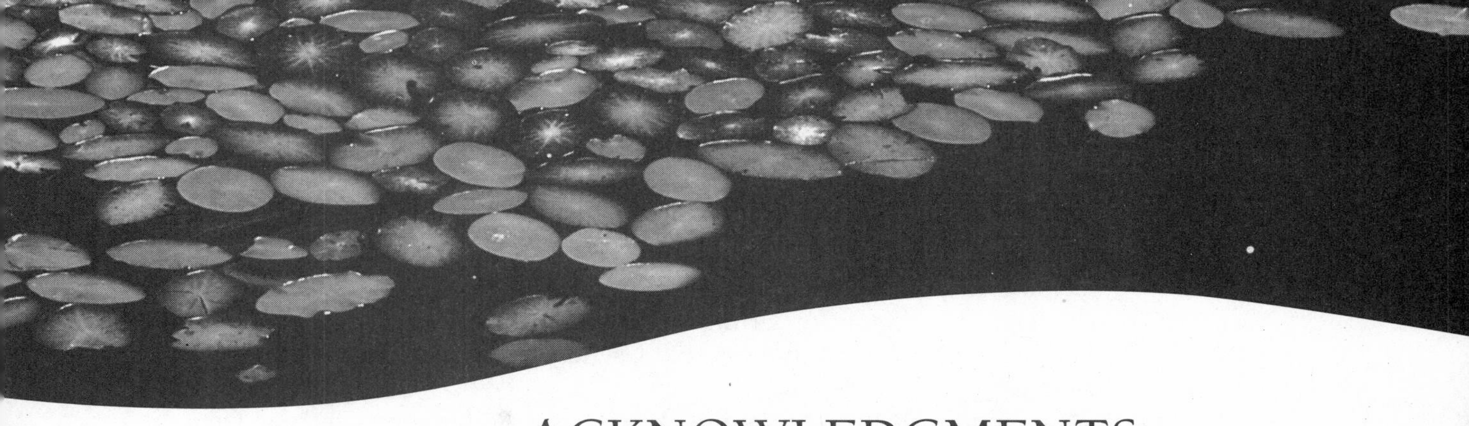

ACKNOWLEDGMENTS

I would like to express my heartfelt thanks to Cynthia and Bob Holzapfel and Warren Jefferson of the Book Publishing Company for believing in this project and all their help with making it happen. A special thanks to Jo Stepaniak for her editing expertise. I am delighted to be part of a project on The Farm, the intentional community in which Book Publishing Company is located and the home of hippie heroes Stephen and Ina May Gaskin.

Mitch Stegall and Christopher Dougherty, you have been such amazing blessings in my life, sharing your lives with my daughters, Sunflower and Rainbeau. Light and Bryan Miller, you always inspire me. Arnel Lindgren, Josie Maran, Jillian Speare, Joe Bob Bruggeman, Janet Yang and Yahn, Jennifer Ogden, David and Steve Karr, Lilakoi Moon, and Bob Ramey, thank you so much for showing up in so many ways in our lives. Jasmine Spring and Andee Smits, I am so grateful for who you are, you stars.

Tamara Kerner, Mindy Green, Martina Hoffmann, Cynthia, Pileggi, Matthew Becker, Anama Star, Marjy Berkman, Kate and Tony Bullings, Farida Sharan, Donna Eagle, Earthstar, Swan Palermo, Gretchen Grace, Midori Gottlieb, Patty Raine, Rondha Baker, the Boulder Raw Group, Debra St. Claire, Laura Lamun, Anne Ward, John Hay, Jennifer Cook and Mo Siegel, Theya and Steve McIntosh, Robert Venosa, Paula Thompson, Jean Marie Swalm, Alana Cini, and Richard Rose, you are my true friends eternally. Many thanks for wise counsel to my friends and colleagues Susun Weed, Rebecca Luna of Rebecca's Apothecary, Camille King, Glynnis Crowley, and the late and great Jeannine Parvati Baker and Rosemary Woodruff Leary.

My dear and beautiful sisters, Dominique Roberts and Rachel Tufunga, I send you much, much love, peace, and prosperity. Thanks Mom and Dad for everything.

Garlic Queen sisters, the way cool herbal sorority, know how I love you! Most of you have gotten so famous you don't need last names! Rosemary, Diana, Rosita, Pam, Beth, Kathi, Cascade, Sara, Linda, and Chanchal.

Best always to my wonderful godchildren, Rosie Ward, Cedar Miller, Aaron Boyleston, James Hay, and Ian and Peter McIntosh.

Thanks to my beautiful husband of over thirty years, Tom Pfeiffer, for true inner and outer beauty and wisdom.

Donovan, you and your musical lyrics have inspired my life. Peter Himmelman, thank you for writing a song about me. Terrence McKenna and William LeSassier, you are both herbal legends, and I am grateful for the time we shared.

Dear goddesses Eve, Aphrodite, Venus, Isis, Persephone, Innana, Diana, Lakshmi, Parvati, Mary, and the many names of love and beauty, thank you. We celebrate you every day in every way. Thank you for coming to visit our planet. We are dedicated in the highest name to healing the earth and making it and ourselves more beautiful and bountiful.

Thank you, God. Thank you, Universe. Blessed be!

All truth—material, philosophic, or spiritual—is both beautiful and good. All real beauty—material art or spiritual symmetry—is both true and good. All genuine goodness—whether personal morality, social equity, or divine ministry—is equally true and beautiful. Health, sanity, and happiness are integrations of truth, beauty, and goodness as they are blended in human experience.

—*The Urantia Book*

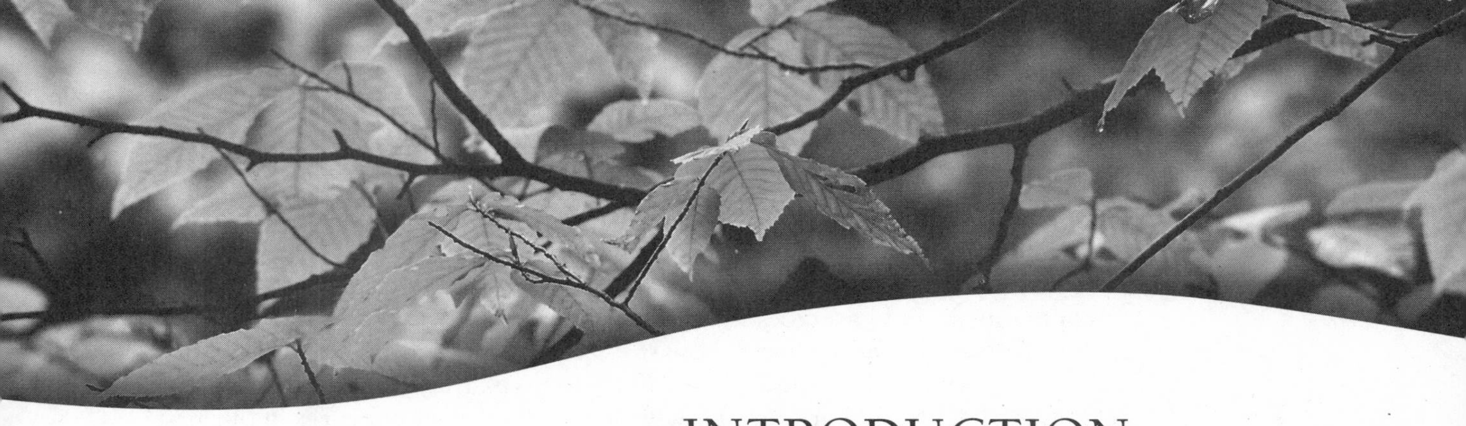

INTRODUCTION
Inner Beauty

Welcome with warm greetings to *Beauty by Nature*!

Beauty gives pleasure to the senses. We marvel at a beautiful sunset, travel miles to take in the wonders of a spacious mountain range or crystalline beach, and marvel at beautiful art. About 90 percent of a first impression is visual and made in the first ten seconds of an encounter, though not all beauty is visual. Babies light up at the presence of a pleasant face. Ancient Greeks would sometimes spare their enemies if they found them exceptionally beautiful. When we are around vital people we feel happier. Beauty is a thing to behold!

It is my desire that this book will help you to become the healthiest and most beautiful you have ever been, inside and out. Our being, though partially expressed through genetics, is also affected by what we think, eat, and how we care for our bodies—these living light temples. It is commonly known that anger can redden skin, fear can pale it, and joy and love can make us radiant. Part of what contributes to our beauty is *chi*, or *prana*, the life force that courses through our beings. *Chi* is the source of energy that promotes warmth, circulation, immunity, metabolism, and digestion. Radiate truth, beauty, and goodness to all you encounter on this dance of life. Be blessed with beauty.

The word "cosmetic" comes from the Greek word *kosmos*, meaning "order in the universe," a concept discussed by the philosopher Pythagoras in 550 BC. It was believed that people who had talents in *kosmetics* were in harmony with their environment, and that if people purified their inner domain, their outer beauty would be enhanced. A *kosmetiko* was someone who was "skilled in adornment." Hence the word "cosmetic."

For thousands of years, millions of people have relied on the bounty of plant preparations to feed, nourish, and cleanse their bodies. Using a shampoo containing lavender or rosemary ensures that somewhere on the face of the earth these plants are growing, blowing, and flowing. Cosmetics that are made in harmony with nature can have a positive effect on our planet. What we apply on our bodies will soon be in our bodies and water systems. We absorb about 60 percent of whatever is put on our skin.

I invite you to awaken and invoke the blessings of natural beauty. A look of contentment and ease goes along with true beauty. Create beauty in every aspect of your life. We've all seen how stress contributes to aging, loss of beauty, and disease. Beautiful people are more likely to take care of themselves, and this encourages health and harmony. How well we take care of ourselves in our first twenty years influences how we will look the rest of our lives. But it's never too late to begin, or begin again.

Let this book be a joyful companion on your evolutionary adventure. You are in charge of what you may or may not need from this book. Share the rest with others. Let self-love and health be the main motivations for becoming your most beautiful self, rather than simply losing weight or having a clearer complexion. No amount of makeup or beauty techniques can camouflage for long an inner being that is less than whole. Delve into the cause of your beauty concerns. Rather than seek out a cream to get rid of acne or puffiness under your eyes, find out what has caused the problem and make changes.

Look in the mirror to see how you are normally perceived by others. Smile. Breathe. Relax. Close your eyes for a few moments and envision yourself as you wish to be. Imagine the scents, textures, and sounds associated with this. Feeling what you want to experience is the first step toward making it happen. When exercising, visualize the type of body you are creating. Allow your baths to be healing and nurturing. When putting lotions on your skin, acknowledge your loving touch and the healing power of the products you are using. Wash your hair lovingly. When eating, say a blessing, and imagine your beautiful food nourishing every cell of your being. Daily, look into your eyes in the mirror and affirm that you love and accept yourself right now. Breathe deeply. Find some time to relax daily.

Starting a Journal

To get the most from this book, I encourage you to have a companion notebook or journal. Use it to write about your goals and concerns as you chart your course to achieving all that you want. Here are some topics to consider writing about in your companion journal.

- Write down ten qualities you appreciate about yourself. Thank your body and all that is right with it. (For example, you might state that you are grateful for your vision, ability to sing, or whatever else serves you.)

- Write down seven aspects of yourself that you would like to improve.
- Take off your clothes in a warm room and have a good look at yourself from all angles. What do you see? What would you like to see? Look in the mirror and imagine a reversal of how you are normally seen by others.
- Write down a dozen things you will do to improve yourself.
- Describe your skin quality. What aspects of your life negatively affect your skin, such as lack of sleep, too many fats or sugars, not enough water, and so forth?
- Weigh yourself and write down your weight. Then write down what you would like to weigh.
- Take your measurements and record them. What do you want your measurements to be in six months (or whatever time frame you choose to reach your goal)?
- What would you enjoy doing if you felt more vital?
- What brings you joy?
- List at least seven pleasures in your life.
- Write down the names of ten people who have influenced your life and how they have helped you grow or change.
- Make a list of your favorite beauty products, and write a few words about why you like them.
- What vices would you like to let go of? Set a date for when you will release them.
- Write about your health history.
- Make a list of five foods you would be better off giving up.
- What is the alternative to your health and beauty concerns? Drugs? Surgery? What will they cost on every level? What will the alternative cost?
- What emotions are you carrying that need to be cleansed?
- Record your thoughts and dreams in your journal.
- Make up your own journal topics! Share your heart.

Affirmations

Pay attention to how you talk. Do any of these sound like you? *I can't. I should. I shouldn't. I hope.* If so, turn these mantras around! *I can! It's an opportunity. I know. I will. I intend. Next time. I deserve to be happy. I can learn from my mistakes. I am confident. I trust in the universe.*

Examples of Affirmations

- Every day I am growing more radiantly beautiful and healthy.
- I consciously make the right choices to become the healthiest and most beautiful person I can be.
- Everything I choose to eat adds to my health, beauty, and attractiveness.
- Food nourishes my being and flows through me.
- I am good to myself.
- I am good to others.
- I am grateful for all the help and blessings that are in my life.
- My body is beautiful and ageless.
- My eyes see clearly.
- My ears hear clearly.
- My mind is alert.
- My skin is radiant and clear.
- I smell pleasant.
- My heart pumps effortlessly.
- My lungs feed me oxygen.
- I sleep soundly.
- I awaken refreshed and rejuvenated.
- I appreciate all the help I have in growing healthier, wiser, more beautiful, and more attractive each day.

Of course, you can create your own affirmations, depending on what your needs are.

Optimistic suggestions will eventually penetrate your consciousness and disempower any negative thoughts. Even if you don't believe your affirmations at first, continuing to say them will help you realize them even sooner. Better yet, write them down and post them where you will see them often. Either way, it's free!

Flower Essences for Inner Beauty

Flower essences are a type of energy or vibrational medicine that can have a subtle, yet beneficial effect on the emotional body. Flower essences are often made by soaking flowers in spring water for several hours, then bottling the water. They can also be purchased in natural food stores and natural apothecaries. Here are a few Bach Flower Essences, developed by Dr. Edward Bach (1886–1936), that can help support you emotionally on your path to radiant beauty.

- **Agrimony** helps reveal the inner and hidden self.
- **Cherry plum** helps release destructive behaviors and relieves tension. It also supports self-discipline.
- **Crab apple** assists with overcoming feelings of uncleanliness and encourages a more positive outlook.
- **Gentian** builds confidence, fortitude, and perseverance so you can succeed.
- **Walnut** eases transitions in life, like relationship changes and moving, but it also helps with dietary changes and letting go of old habits.

To use flower essences, simply put two drops of the remedy into a glass of spring water and sip it throughout the day. Flower essences can aid in your transformation, should any of the above remedies sound like something you need. It is fine to mix up to six different ones together.

Though it may seem overwhelming and time-consuming to do the rituals that help us become our most beautiful selves, it is so worthwhile. One suggestion is to make a list of all of the practices you feel would benefit your well-being. Your list might be long or short and could include a variety of possibilities: simple dietary changes, such as drinking lemon juice in water; exercise, such as yoga or the Tibetan Five Rites (see page 158); or beauty treatments, such as aromatherapy baths, facial acupressure (see page 90), or facial masks. Write the days of the week across the top of the page, then make copies. Use this chart to track at least seven healthful and beautifying techniques daily.

Enjoy the adventure of transforming into your most beautiful self. May we all live in beauty, abundance, and health on every level!

Blessed Be. Om Shanti,
Brigitte Mars

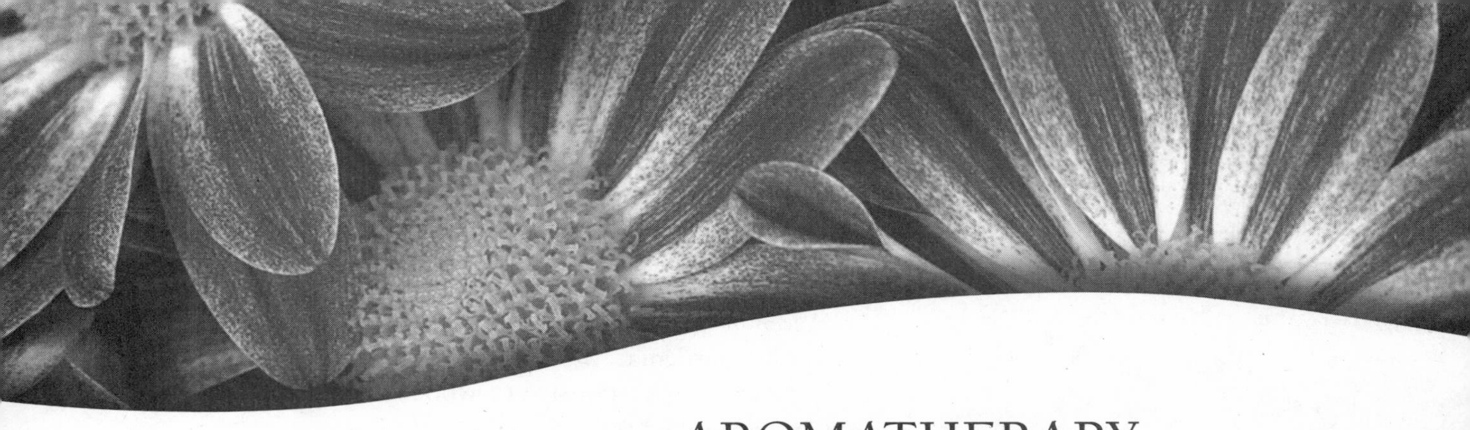

AROMATHERAPY
Getting Started with Beauty by Nature

Aromatherapy is the practice of using essential plant oils for healing body, mind, and spirit. Many essential oils are suggested throughout this book to help you care for your body, promote healing, and enhance your beauty.

One of the most ancient methods of aromatherapy was to burn aromatic branches and inhale the smoke. The word "perfume" is derived from the Latin *per fumum*, meaning "through smoke." Nowadays natural food stores carry a selection of aromatherapy diffusers that range from simple plug-in devices to test-tube appliances and those powered by candles. It is lovely and more healthful to enjoy plant fragrances and their therapeutic values without smoke.

Essential oils help protect plants from fungi and viruses. They also help repel predator insects and attract beneficial pollinators. Essential oils do not contain pollens, but in some cases they can trigger allergenic or sneezing reactions in some sensitive individuals. Essential oils, also known as volatile oils, are distilled or pressed from plants, flowers, or food. Their fragrance reaches our nose, is taken into the air we breathe, and eventually goes into our bloodstream. Scent travels along a neurological pathway, bypassing the blood-brain barrier. When essential oils are smelled, they can stimulate neurotransmitter production.

Essential oils are believed to interrupt the oxygenation cycles of bacteria and interact with the receptor sites in the central nervous system. Essential oils kill germs, bacteria, fungi, and viruses, but not friendly intestinal flora. Bacteria do not appear to grow resistant to essential oils.

Essential oils are liposoluble, which means they are able to penetrate the skin and travel through the bloodstream and interstitial fluids. Many oils (for example, anise, eucalyptus, fennel, and sage) contain phytosterols, substances similar to hormones that can positively affect the skin. Essential oils act quickly and are eliminated from the system within two to five hours.

During pregnancy, the only essential oils considered safe enough for topical use are small amounts of the following:

- chamomile
- clary sage
- geranium
- jasmine
- lavender
- neroli
- peppermint
- rose
- rosemary
- ylang-ylang

The following essential oils should *always be avoided during pregnancy:*

- angelica
- anise
- basil
- bitter almond
- camphor
- cinnamon
- clary sage
- clove
- cypress
- fennel
- frankincense
- hyssop
- juniper
- lovage
- marjoram
- myrrh
- oregano
- pennyroyal
- rosemary
- sage
- sassafras
- savory
- thyme
- wintergreen

Humans are said to have an estimated ten million cells for detecting scents. It has been said that the nose is the gateway to the brain. Our sense of smell is our most primitive sense, and what we smell can affect our health and consciousness.

Women often prefer floral smells that evoke pleasant memories: gardenia, rose, and jasmine, for example. Men seem to be most responsive to woodsy, citrus, and spicy scents, like cinnamon and ginger.

Quality is imperative. Be sure you are using pure essential plant oils and not synthetic fragrances. Synthetic fragrances are likely allergenic culprits in many cosmetics. Though you might not be able to tell the difference, your body will. Be suspicious of clear bottles and companies where each essential oil is the same price, as these are most likely fragrances, not pure essential oils and not necessarily natural or therapeutic. Absolutes and resins are likely to contain chemicals and should never be used internally. For that matter, avoid ingesting essential oils at all, unless you have taken a class or really learned more about the subject, as they are very concentrated and can be toxic if ingested improperly.

To obtain one-third ounce of marjoram essential oil, it takes 6.6 pounds of the herb; for clary sage to yield one-third ounce of essential oil, 8.8 pounds are needed. For rosemary, 22 pounds of the herb are required for one-third ounce of essential oil; and as much as 1,100 pounds of roses are needed for one-third ounce of rose essential oil. Essential oils are very concentrated. One drop is equal to about one teaspoon of the dried spice. Essential oils require lots of resources to generate—use ecologically.

Tips for Using Essential Oils

- Keep essential oils out of the reach of children and away from light, heat, plastics, and metals. Some oils can stain clothing and damage the finish on furniture.
- It is best to smell essential oils in a well-ventilated area, as headaches and nausea can result from too much exposure.
- Add a drop of essential oil to a tablespoon of water. If it appears slick and milky, there may be synthetics added.

- Keep essential oils away from mucous membranes, such as the eyes, mouth, and genitals, as well as broken skin.
- Place a drop of essential oil on a scrap of paper. If an oil stain still is apparent two hours later, the essential oil may have been diluted with vegetable oils.
- Refrigerate citrus oils, as they have a shelf life of only about a year.
- Those with high blood pressure should avoid essential oils of hyssop, rosemary, sage, and thyme, or use only very small amounts.
- Those with epilepsy should avoid essential oils of fennel, hyssop, sage, and thuja.
- When using essential oils for children, use half the amount.
- If you have any doubts about the safety of an essential oil, avoid it.

Most essential oils are too strong to use alone; they should be diluted in a good-quality, cold-pressed carrier oil. Some of my favorite carrier oils are almond, grapeseed, and apricot kernel oil, because they are light and don't have a strong smell. Sometimes a stronger oil, such as hazelnut or sesame, is preferred, particularly when creating a more warming blend. Jojoba, which is technically a wax, is excellent for creating products intended for dry skin. Essential oils can also be diluted in warm water. Lavender and tea tree essential oils are some of the few oils that are safe to use undiluted.

Be sure to use a different pipette or dropper for each essential oil you measure out. Dipping the same hollow tube into different bottles can cause cross contamination.

Aromatherapy doesn't have to be complicated; it can be as simple as smelling the flowers. Take a workshop in aromatherapy to learn more about this ancient fragrant art. Let the blessings of botanicals enhance your natural beauty.

Some essential oils are considered toxic and should not be used without guidance from a qualified aromatherapist. These oils include the following:

- anise
- bay
- camphor
- hyssop
- lemongrass
- mugwort
- pennyroyal
- sage
- sassafras
- savory
- tarragon
- thyme
- wintergreen
- wormwood

Beauty by Nature

CHAPTER 1

A Beautiful State of Mind by Nature

BEAUTIFUL MIND

Give me beauty in the inward soul; and may the inner and outer be at one.

—ANONYMOUS

Outer beauty certainly begins within. Think positively. Look for the good qualities and similarities we have with each other, rather than getting hung up on our differences.

Dispel negative thoughts such as jealousy, anger, and worry by journaling, talking to a trusted friend, and trying to find the lessons and opportunities for growth in all the difficulties that come into your life. I sometimes ask myself, "Now what am I supposed to learn from this experience?"

We could all benefit from clearer thinking. Though the brain makes up only about 2 percent of our total body weight, it requires about 20 percent of the body's total oxygen intake. Breathing more deeply and slowly nourishes the brain with oxygen, which can literally "feed our head." The left brain corresponds to linear thought, such as language and logic. The right brain corresponds more to spatial functions, such as imagination and intuition.

High-chlorophyll foods are excellent oxygen transporters, and "superfoods" like wheatgrass, barley-grass juice, and blue-green algae can help one think more clearly. Other high-chlorophyll foods include leafy greens such as kale, collards, and beet greens. Sea vegetables have traditionally been used to increase longevity and clear thinking. Select foods that are fresh and unprocessed. High-carbohydrate foods also affect thinking. Concentrated sources of carbs such as potatoes, pasta, rice, bread, and other forms of grain tend to make us feel mentally serene rather than sharp. Lots of carbs at lunch, such as bread or pasta, can leave you less productive for the afternoon. Heated fats make us feel foggy, soggy, and groggy, and along with free radicals, they combine in the bloodstream to produce a waste product called *lipofuscin*, which can adversely affect brain function. Brains rely on a constant stream of nutrients, blood sugar, and oxygen to produce the energy that facilitates learning, thoughts, and actions. Sugar causes our bodies to lose valuable nutrients.

Protect your brain by avoiding aluminum, claimed by many health authorities to be cumulative in the brain and contributing to Alzheimer's disease. Aluminum cookware, tinfoil, nondairy coffee creamers, commercial baking powders, and many deodorants (which get absorbed through the lymph nodes under the arms) can accumulate and cause lesions in the brain and reduce vitamin C levels. Chemical exposure through items such as housecleaning products, pesticides, paints, and some art supplies and cosmetics can affect the brain adversely. Researchers believe that mercury toxicity (such as from silver dental fillings) can be a factor in Alzheimer's disease.

Herbs for a Beautiful Mind

Herbs have been used throughout history to improve mental capacity. Here are a few good choices.

- **Bacopa** is a nervine and memory enhancer that improves neurotransmitter function and increases serotonin levels.
- **Eleuthero**, formerly known as Siberian ginseng, is nourishing to the pituitary and adrenal glands. It helps the body's ability to deal with stress. Studies done in the former Soviet Union show that this herb helps to improve job accuracy.
- **Gotu kola** has been used in India as a cerebral and endocrine tonic. Containing calcium and phosphorus as well as the amino acid glutamine, this renowned herb has been used to treat amnesia, dementia, fatigue, and senility. It has a revitalizing effect on the brain cells and nerves.
- **Ginkgo** improves the brain's ability to utilize oxygen and glucose by improving peripheral blood flow. Ginkgo has been found to improve nerve

signal transmission and activate adenosine troposphere (ATP), an organic compound that aids metabolic reactions. Ginkgo helps protect nerve cells from free radical damage. It is an antioxidant and cerebral tonic.

- **Reishi mushrooms** promote mental clarity and peacefulness.
- **Rosemary** has a delightful aroma and long European tradition of alleviating anxiety. Ancient Greek scholars wore laurels of rosemary when taking examinations to improve memory.
- **Licorice** is sweet and energizing, improves vitality, and helps keep blood sugar levels stable. Licorice is a *chi* tonic, nutritive and rejuvenative.
- **Oat straw** and **milky oat seed** are rich in calcium and silica and nourish the nervous system. They are considered cerebral and nerve tonics, nutritive and rejuvenative.
- Aromas that can be used to stimulate mental alertness include **basil, lemon, lemongrass, lime, peppermint,** and **rosemary essential oils.** It is ideal to smell such aromas when studying and then use them again when taking a test or having to perform.
- **Chamomile, lavender,** and **neroli essential oils** stimulate serotonin production, thus calming fear, anxiety, stress, and insomnia.

Brain Power

The old man keeps all his mental powers so long as he gives up neither using them nor adding to them.

—CICERO

The brain is an organ that gains strength with the balance of repose and right use. You may find the following techniques helpful for improving mental ability.

- Expand your experiences. Even the simple act of traveling to work by new routes can inspire different thoughts as you see new things.
- Sharpen your senses by really focusing. Notice as many details as possible. Experience with as many senses as possible.
- Absentmindedness means that the mind was not present or focusing on the matters at hand. “Be here now” truly is good advice.
- Practice good posture to improve the flow of energy throughout the nervous system.
- Exercise to increase your intake of oxygen. This speeds up nerve impulses between brain cells. Working up a sweat three times a week is important. Dance!

- Read things that are challenging and that give new insights. Read the classics. Enjoy a genre that you have never before read such as autobiographies, science fiction, or history.
- Color therapists say that the color yellow is cerebrally stimulating. Highlight important passages that you read in yellow, wear yellow clothing and accessories, and visualize breathing in the color. Consider using yellow in lighting and decor in places where mental work is being done.
- Quietly and closely, observe nature. She abounds with beauty and intelligence, even in minute detail that can inspire us in a positive way.
- Always have a pen and paper available. Write down details: phone numbers, tasks to do, and goals. Getting things out of your mind and onto paper will help free you up for more creative endeavors. Keep an engagement calendar. Record your flashes of brilliance and words of wisdom! It will help you put them to use. Make lists into meaningful categories.
- When you want to remember something, repeat it aloud to yourself. Visualize it being imprinted upon your brain.
- Think positively. You'll probably do better if you affirm that "I can pass this exam" rather than "I'll never make it."
- Avoid damaging substances such as cigarettes, alcohol, pollutants, artificial sweeteners, and MSG. Some medications have an adverse effect on the brain.
- Creative people usually retain a childlike quality. Be willing to play. Draw.
- The art of visualization is one way of practicing mental gymnastics. Einstein supposedly came upon the theory of relativity while visualizing flying along at the speed of light.
- Be aware that trauma, food allergies, yeast overgrowth, addiction, and nutritional deficiencies can all contribute to impairment of the intellect and memory loss.
- Introverts tend to have their most creative time in the early morning, while extroverts do better at night.
- Keep your things organized. Get rid of clutter and distractions. Learn about feng shui.

Learn to Meditate

Meditate to become more relaxed, intuitive, gain expanded awareness, and attain a more youthful appearance. Meditation helps counteract stress, focuses the mind, slows down the heart, lowers blood pressure, quiets mental chatter, and helps us live more fully in the present.

To meditate, sit comfortably, cross-legged or on a straight-backed chair with your feet touching the floor. Close your eyes. Your mind may fill with chatter. Allow the thoughts to come and just drift past, like watching a movie. Avoid thinking or rationalizing what the images mean. Just let the movie roll. Breathe deeply.

You may want to learn to meditate by focusing on your "third eye" or using a mantra such as "om," "Jesus," or "peace." You can also meditate with a single candle made of beeswax, hempseed oil, or soybean wax on an altar. Focus on the flame and clear your mind of thoughts. Or have a beautiful mandala picture to gaze upon. I am partial to the Shri Yantra.

Meditation is ideally practiced twice daily, at dawn and dusk for about twenty minutes each session.

- Learn new skills: language, musical instrument, dance, martial arts, or drawing. Take a class at a local community college. Join a book club.
- Keep an open heart and open mind. Keep learning your entire life. Be open to the possibilities . . .

BREATHING IN BEAUTY

In Sanskrit, *pranayama* is considered the science of breath. *Prana* is the life force that permeates our beings. When we breathe more fully and deeply, we become more aware, more intuitive, calmer, alert, and have an integration of body, mind, and spirit. Breathing deeply massages the internal organs, increasing circulation and bringing nutrients to all parts of the body.

Inhale through your nose to filter out particulates and more directly stimulate the brain. Repressing breathing can repress feelings. There is a common lineage shared among the words "spirit," "inspiration," and "respiration." Oxygen nourishes every cell in our being.

The lungs expand and contract about twenty thousand times a day. The average person draws in twelve breaths a minute. This process brings oxygen and *prana* into the body and eliminates carbon dioxide. Through our lungs we are directly connected to our environment.

It takes about one minute for blood to circulate through the body and return to the heart. Our lungs can hold up to seven pints of air when fully expanded, yet most people only take in a pint of air with each breath, which makes the diaphragm stiff and causes us to feel rigid and uptight. When our breathing is shallow, our heart rate quickens and stress levels increase. The mind helps control the breath, which helps control the blood. Breathing more deeply causes energy to rise and increases our sensory perception.

On an emotional level, the lungs correlate to the emotion of grief. Crying and other forms of self-expression can clear our lungs of stored emotions that can make us prone to lung weakness. Fatigue is sometimes caused by a lack of oxygen in our cells.

As we age, our breathing tends to get shallower. People with weak lungs often speak in a monotone and may sound like there is sorrow in their voices. Laughter and exercise bring fresh oxygen into the lungs and help to clean them; they also increase energy! Playing a musical instrument and singing are great ways to increase respiratory capacity. Stand tall; good posture improves lung capacity. Let fresh air into your home.

Foods that nourish the lungs include green and yellow foods that are high in beta-carotene like winter squashes, pumpkin, kale and collards, carrots, bell peppers, turnips, apples, cherries, and peaches. Chlorophyll, found in greens, is extremely nourishing. The pungent foods onions, scallions, garlic, cayenne, ginger, horseradish, daikon, and mustard greens all help to disperse lung congestion.

The color orange benefits the lungs; visualize breathing it in. Wear amber, coral, and/or topaz.

Sallow, pale, and puffy cheeks may indicate weak, underactive lungs. Pimples on the cheeks may indicate lung toxicity, and pale cheeks may be a sign of excess dairy consumption. Lung disorders can manifest as skin problems, loss of body hair, frequent colds, or phlegm.

Breathing Exercises

How we breathe can affect our health, beauty, and consciousness. Breathing through your nose warms the air and helps to trap microbes and particles before they reach your lungs. It is better to breathe into your belly rather than breathing only into your chest. When we inhale it is good to visualize taking in life force, and as we exhale, let go of tensions and toxins. Or visualize that you are the ocean and your breath is the waves. Breathe deeply and fully, and do your best to make the exhale longer than the inhale. Practice deep breathing exercises daily.

Yoga Breathing

Yoga breathing helps us have better control over our lungs. Inhale deeply for a count of five, allowing your chest and belly to expand. Hold for a count of five (unless you have high blood pressure). Inhale a sniff of air. Exhale slowly to a count of five, relaxing your shoulders and pulling your belly inward. Repeat seven times. Visualize your breath traveling up your spine and down the front of your body.

Deep Relaxation Breath

Lie on the floor with a pillow supporting your knees. Place your palms over your abdomen, with your fingers gently laced just above your navel. Breathe in to a count of three as your abdomen pushes your fingers toward the ceiling. Exhale to a count of five as your fingers and abdomen move toward the floor.

The Complete Breath

1. Lie down in a quiet place with your arms at your sides, palms down. Close your eyes and slowly inhale through your nose as your abdomen expands. Pull the air up into your rib cage and finally into your chest.

Hold the breath for a few seconds. Breathe out slowly while drawing in your abdomen and relaxing your chest and rib cage.

2. Breathe in again slowly as in step 1, but raise your arms above your head until the backs of your hands touch the floor. Stretch and hold for ten seconds. As you slowly exhale, bring your arms back to your sides.
3. Repeat steps 1 and 2 several times.

Aromatherapy for Better Breathing

Essential oils that benefit the lungs when used as aromatherapy (not ingested) include eucalyptus, ginger, lavender (the best one for kids), marjoram, peppermint, pine, rosemary, sage, tea tree, and thyme.

Aromatherapy Inhaler

Here is a simple remedy to brighten your mood and invigorate your energy; it will also calm you down during the day. To make an aromatherapy nasal inhaler, add 5 drops essential oil (basil, lavender, rosemary, or eucalyptus are all excellent) to 1/4 teaspoon Celtic sea salt. Place the ingredients in a small glass vial with a lid. Open and inhale up to ten deep breaths at a time.

CHAPTER 2

Beautiful Skin by Nature

HEALTHY SKIN

Our skin is our interface with the world and corresponds to our inner processes. Skin protects us and mirrors our health. It has a multitude of functions: sensory device, excretory and respiratory organ, and temperature regulator. Skin protects the bones and organs of the body by keeping them clean and holding them in place. Our skin is our largest organ, weighing about seven to ten pounds and covering about twenty square feet. This amazing covering is supplied with more nerve endings than any other organ except the brain. The average square inch of skin can contain 65 hairs, 650 sweat glands, 100 sebaceous glands, 78 heat sensors, 13 cold sensors, 10,000 cells, 1,300 nerve endings, 19 yards of blood vessels, 78 yards of nerves, and 165 separate pressure-sensing structures, enabling us to sense pleasure, pain, pressure, and hot and cold temperatures. Skin also provides a direct link to the brain and every other portion of the nervous system. Our skin can store up to 44 pounds of fat and up to 22 pounds of water. It is our most resilient organ. Skin is thinnest on our eyelids and thickest on the soles of our feet.

The French have a saying for people who are confident: *bien dans sa peau*, which literally means they "feel good in their skin." The skin is referred to as our "third lung" in Asian medicine, and its health is governed by the lungs and large intestine and, to a lesser degree, the blood, kidneys, and liver. Some refer to skin as a "second brain." Skin discriminates, communicates, and receives love. We pale when fearful, blush when embarrassed, and glow when delighted. Whatever happens to the skin often corresponds to something going on inside the mind and body. When dealing with skin problems, ask what the skin is trying to tell you on an emotional level. For example, blemishes may serve to protect us from the threat of intimacy or signify that we may want to "jump out of our skin." If you are dealing with skin problems, do your best to understand what was going on in your life at the time they started. Dermatologists feel that at least one-third of skin diseases are psychosomatic in nature. To have beautiful, irresistible skin, learn to touch and nurture yourself.

All of our negative emotions, problems, and harmful habits are mirrored in our skin. On the other hand, our skin can also reflect joy, love, a healthful diet, and the positive effects of exercise.

About 2 percent of the oxygen that enters the body does so through the skin. Toxins are released from the body through the skin in the form of perspiration. About 20 percent of the body's elimination occurs through perspiration; both the skin and kidneys help eliminate toxins. When the kidneys are not functioning optimally, the skin has to work harder.

The skin is also a major producer of endocrine hormones, which govern the sensation of touch and connect the skin to every cell and organ throughout its vast network of nerves. Skin is constantly exposed to the external environment more directly than any other organ.

The skin has seven cell layers. The thin outer layer is the epidermis, which is the part of the skin that is visible and gets touched. The epidermis is about .05 inches thick and is primarily made up of several layers of collagen and elastin.

The epidermis protects against bacteria, viruses, and sun damage. New skin cells are regenerated from within, moving upward to the top outer layer, or stratum corneum. Immature cells below the surface need this protective layer to keep them healthy as they develop. By the time they reach the stratum corneum, the cells are elongated, dried out, and dead; eventually they are sloughed off. Cellular renewal takes about twenty-eight

Factors That Can Affect Our Skin

- Sleep (quantity and quality)
- Emotions (joy and love as well as sadness, stress, fear, and grief)
- Hormones
- Cigarette smoke
- Diet
- Quality of drinking water
- Sun exposure
- Scrubbing the skin
- Cosmetics
- Swimming in chlorinated water
- Chemicals in soap, bubble baths, lotions, and dry cleaning fluid residue
- Chemicals in tap water
- Chemical contact (such as with cleaning products, art supplies, and conventional beauty products)
- Medications
- Physically demanding work that exposes the skin to sun, wind, and/or heat
- Loss of moisture that doesn't get replenished
- Constipation
- Poor oxygen intake (lack of fresh air, stuffy rooms, air pollution)

days; fourteen of these days are required for the new cells to make it to the surface, where they live for about another fourteen days, after which they are rubbed off or fall off and are replaced by other mature cells. Amazingly, our skin repairs itself after an injury. The older we get, the longer it takes for new cells to replace worn-out ones, which can take up to sixty days. Epidermal renewal is most pronounced between midnight and 4:00 a.m., when other body systems are at rest. It's another good reason to sleep at night!

The epidermis also contains about half of the body's leukocytes, a type of white blood cell. Also in the epidermis are melanocytes, which are skin cells that contain the pigment melanin, which gives the skin color, allows it to tan, and helps protect it from the sun. People with darker skin have more melanin.

The topmost epidermal cells are covered with an oily, waterproof film, or hydrolipid barrier, that helps the skin retain water. Many modern high-tech skin care regimes can destroy this protective barrier.

Beneath the epidermis is the dermis, or corium, which is composed of collagen and elastin protein fibers woven together to form a threadlike network. In the dermis, there are also fat cells, which provide insulation against cold, and a network of lymphatic endings and capillaries, as well as nerve endings that carry pleasure and pain reception. They are all nestled in a supportive system of collagen and elastin, which holds the skin together and gives it resiliency and the ability to stretch and regain its shape. There are three types of protein in the skin, which account for about 30 percent of the skin's composition. Keratin is found in the epidermis, and collagen and elastin are in the dermis and connective tissue. As we get older, the cross-connections of these filaments, which originally ran parallel to each other and used to allow more room for circulation, become more matted (frequent exposure to hot water is one factor).

The sebaceous glands next to the hair shafts provide both the hair and skin with sebum, which helps protect the skin and scalp against drying out. There are about 300,000 sebaceous glands that produce about .07 ounces of sebum a day. If the ends of the sebaceous glands become congested, pimples, blackheads, and skin infections can occur. Excess sebum can be a factor in acne. Hormonal changes, including puberty, menstruation, and foods that contain or stimulate estrogen, can cause excess sebum production. If there is not enough sebum, dryness will be the result. Water makes up over 70 percent of the content of our skin (about the same percentage as our planet). As we age, our skin will contain less water, closer to 60 percent.

The skin is constantly being replaced with cells that originate in the hair follicles. Our skin may get clogged from the interior (due to congesting food or ingested toxins, for example) or the exterior (from dirt, chemicals, or cosmetics). When the epidermis gets clogged with excess dead cells, toxins, sweat, and/or sebum, pimples and whiteheads can erupt. When hair follicles become encrusted with a buildup of dry skin, keratosis pilaris can occur; this is a skin condition characterized by hard tiny bumps, most commonly on the upper arms and thighs.

Foods for Skin Care

Foods to eat more of to improve skin quality include the dark orange beta-carotene foods like apricots, cantaloupe, peaches, winter squash, carrots, pumpkin, and sweet potatoes. Other foods that nourish the skin include apples, avocados, green leafy vegetables, and parsley. Be sure to include some foods rich in high-quality oils in your diet, such as avocados, hempseeds, raw nuts and seeds, coconut, and extra-virgin olive oil. Blueberries help improve skin disorders (such as eczema and burns), promote collagen production, and help prevent wrinkles. Eat a big green salad daily, and include items like watercress, arugula, mustard greens, cucumbers, radishes, shredded beets, and carrots. Be sure to make your own salad dressing using extra-virgin olive oil.

Drinking at least two quarts of pure water a day is essential. Water helps to eliminate substances that would clog the pores. Adding a squeeze of lemon or lime juice helps the blood stay more fluid. Fresh vegetable juices made from beets, carrots, celery, cucumbers, parsley, and spinach will make your skin glow. It's always a good idea to dilute vegetable and fruit juices with at least equal amounts of water, as they can be very sweet and elevate blood sugar levels. Be aware that alcoholic beverages, caffeine-containing sodas, and coffee can dehydrate the skin.

Foods to avoid for healthier skin include fried foods, refined carbohydrates, wheat products, and heated fats (which includes commercial bottled salad dressings and baked goods). Sugar creates an acid condition leading to skin breakouts. Overeating causes blood to be diverted to the stomach to aid digestion, thus leaving the skin lacking all it deserves.

Herbal Allies for the Skin

- **Aloe vera** is anti-inflammatory and antifungal. It contains biogenic stimulators that promote new cellular growth.
- **Burdock** softens the skin and helps decrease acne, dandruff, eczema, hives, psoriasis, and ringworm.
- **Calendula** increases circulation to peripheral body parts and inhibits pus formation.
- **Chamomile** promotes skin repair and renewal. It relaxes facial muscles and helps repair dry skin and wounds.

- **Chickweed** aids in fat metabolism. It may also be used topically for burns, eczema, itchy skin, psoriasis, rashes, and to help dissolve warts.
- **Cleavers** cleanses the kidneys and thus improves acne, dandruff, eczema, and psoriasis.
- **Comfrey** helps draw infection out of the body. Used topically, it helps heal dry skin, burns, and wounds. Allantoin, one of its constituents, stimulates cell proliferation.
- **Dandelion root tea**, when consumed, revitalizes sallow skin and relieves liver congestion. It is a classic herb to improve acne, boils, eczema, and psoriasis, when taken internally.
- **Echinacea** stimulates macrophage activity and helps regenerate skin. It is used to treat abscesses, acne, boils, eczema, herpes, and insect bites.
- **Elder flowers** help cleanse the pores from the inside out and are used internally to treat acne.
- **Fennel** helps clear liver obstruction and moistens the body. It is used topically in antiwrinkle formulas and lotions.
- **Horsetail's** high mineral content nourishes all aspects of the body's structure. It is an excellent herb to improve acne, eczema, and weak skin in general.
- **Irish moss** softens and moistens skin. It also prevents premature wrinkling and dry skin.
- **Licorice** soothes irritated tissues and helps reduce age spots and herpes sores.
- **Marshmallow root** is mucilaginous and moisturizing for dry skin and irritated tissues. It helps relieve dry scalp, eczema, psoriasis, sunburn, and wounds.
- **Nettle** is a timeless remedy to treat acne, eczema, and psoriasis. It improves circulation, builds the blood, and cleanses the liver and kidneys.
- **Oregon grape root** strengthens the liver and contains infection-fighting properties that deter skin infections. It improves acne, boils, eczema, herpes, psoriasis, and infected wounds.
- **Plantain leaf** clears infection and soothes inflammation and irritated tissues due to its high mucilage content. Used topically, it helps draw out infection and is used to reduce boils, insect bites, and poison ivy.
- **Red clover blossom** helps the body do a better job of cleansing the blood, liver, and lymphatic vessels. It improves acne, eczema, and psoriasis.
- **Violet leaves** speed the healing of acne, boils, eczema, and psoriasis.
- **Vitex berries** help normalize the pituitary gland and hormone production. Vitex is a helpful herb for hormone-related acne and herpes.

- **Witch hazel bark's** high flavonoid content helps heal damaged blood vessels. It is used topically to benefit acne, blemishes, eczema, poison ivy, and sunburn.
- **Yarrow leaves** open the pores and facilitate the elimination of waste material through the skin. Yarrow is used internally and topically for acne and eczema.
- **Yellow dock** helps detoxify the liver and blood and thus improves acne, boils, eczema, jaundice, and psoriasis.

Vitamins for Skin Care

Since good skin health begins from within, various vitamins can be of benefit. Vitamin A and its precursor, beta-carotene, help preserve the skin's elasticity, regulate sebaceous glands, protect against infection, and stimulate collagen formation. A deficiency in this vitamin may result in dry, itchy skin, making it more likely that dead skin cells will clog the pores and cause breakouts. The B-complex vitamins help keep the ravages of stress from showing on our skin. A deficiency is sometimes implicated in cracks around the mouth, corners of the mouth, and eyes. Vitamin C strengthens the capillaries, promotes healing, stimulates collagen production, and increases skin elasticity. Bioflavonoids help keep the capillaries strong, thereby inhibiting bruises, spider veins, and varicose veins. Vitamin D nourishes dry skin. Vitamin E helps the body utilize oxygen better, balances hormone production, and preserves elasticity by preventing collagen breakdown. Vitamin F is often referred to as "the cosmetic vitamin." A deficiency can cause wrinkles, eczema, and thick, dry skin. A deficiency in iron can leave us looking pale and "washed out." Selenium, along with vitamins E and C, helps preserve the skin's elasticity. Zinc helps to synthesize collagen and boost the immune system; it is essential to bringing dry, flaky skin into balance.

Eczema and Psoriasis

Eczema, also known as contact dermatitis, allergic dermatitis, and many other names, can be chronic or temporary and is characterized by abraded, cracked, blistered, weepy, crusted, and/or patchy dry skin along with intense, incessant itching and inflammation; almost anything you touch seems to make it worse. Eczema is most prevalent in autumn and is often worse at night.

Scratching itchy skin can cause more irritation and make you more prone to infection. Consider keeping your fingernails very short and even wearing gloves to sleep in to prevent making things worse.

Psoriasis is a chronic inflammatory skin condition characterized by small scaly silvery pink and red patches commonly occurring on the knees, elbows, chest, scalp, lower back, and buttocks. Psoriasis scales stick to crystalline swellings, and if scraped off may bleed. Psoriasis involves chronic rapidly growing cells (often forming at five to ten times the normal rate) that come to the skin's surface before they are fully mature, at a faster rate than old skin can be shed. The thickened scaly areas of psoriasis do not contain pus or sebum and are unlikely to itch.

Psoriasis is believed to be related to a weakened immune system. Factors that make us more susceptible include diet, alcohol consumption, environmental factors, genetics, infection, problems in lipid metabolism, obesity, smoking, surgery, and trauma. Psoriasis can be mild to disabling and is considered more stubborn than eczema.

As both eczema and psoriasis tend to move around, change, and spread, they are often considered "wind invasion" in Asian medicine. With both ailments it is helpful to cool the blood and skin.

Is stress making you want to claw out of your skin? Then look at what can be done to mellow your lifestyle. Anger, anxiety, fatigue, frustration, grief, and worry can worsen psoriasis or be contributing factors. People who suffer from psoriasis tend to be always on the run, moving rapidly, just like their skin growth. Slow down. Practice stress reduction. Massage is a good way to soothe the tension from the body. Children with skin disorders may benefit from extra cuddling at night before bed.

Chemical and physical irritation (such as rough clothing), metabolic imbalances, stress, and even weather conditions can cause the body to respond by forming a protective barrier. Many culprits can contribute to eczema and psoriasis from the outside. Overly vigorous washing, reactions to soaps, bubble baths, shampoos, hair dyes, lotions, cosmetics, nail polishes, laundry soaps, pet allergies, and chlorinated and overly hot water are common examples. Use fragrance-free products and avoid skin contact with chemicals. Remember that whatever gets on your body can be absorbed by as much as 60 percent by the skin. Don't pollute your body or the planet. By taking care of one, the other will thrive.

Be aware of what you wear. If possible, avoid wearing elastic, nylon, spandex, suede, wool, and fabrics made with synthetic fibers. Dry cleaning fluid residue and synthetic laundry soaps can irritate. It may be helpful to add one cup of apple cider vinegar to the final rinse of a laundry load to neutralize possible irritants.

Climatotherapy indicates that brief exposure to natural sunlight can improve or even clear psoriasis. Eczema tends to react poorly to sunshine and salt water. However, psoriasis seems to recede in their presence. Swimming in the ocean may be helpful to both eczema and psoriasis. Swimming in the Dead Sea is a famous remedy for relieving psoriasis.

Add one pound of baking soda and one cup of apple cider vinegar, or two handfuls of rolled oats tied into a cloth, to your bathwater. You could also add essential oils to your bath. Apply black tea with a clean cloth. The tannic acid in tea helps dry up eczema blisters.

Short, daily exposure to sunlight improves or clears psoriasis for many people. Get plenty of fresh air and exercise to ensure good circulation. Exercise enough to work up a good sweat. Saunas can be a way to clear internal toxins. Practice deep breathing as much as possible. Remember that the lungs and large intestines govern the skin in Asian medicine.

If more infants were breast-fed, it would help cut down on the amount of eczema and psoriasis. However, it is possible that a nursing babe who has eczema or psoriasis (or many other conditions) could have allergies to a food the mom is consuming, so the mom may need to alter her diet somewhat to eliminate the possible harmful agents. Food allergies are often the main cause of eczema and/or psoriasis. Both are considered inflammatory conditions. What reduces inflammation? Enzymes! Where are they found? In fresh raw foods! So often we crave the food or foods we are allergic to. That may be the main causative factor in most people's skin disorders. Find out what is causing your inflammation and eliminate it. Foods to avoid include heated chocolate, dairy products, citrus juice, tomatoes, meat, eggs, peanut butter, potatoes, wheat products, soy foods, fried foods, food additives, and hydrogenated and heated oils (which includes most bottled salad dressings). Any food allergen can be a contributing factor to a skin condition. Eat plenty of green leafy vegetables. Drink a diluted vegetable juice daily made from celery, cucumbers, beets, and parsley. Use extra-virgin olive oil as your main fat. Include three tablespoons of freshly ground flaxseeds daily, or learn to make flaxseed crackers. Taking raw organic hempseed oil might be helpful.

A tea or extract taken three times daily made with burdock root, calendula, chickweed, cleavers, raw dandelion root, nettle leaf, Oregon grape root, plantain leaf, prickly ash bark, red clover blossoms, Saint John's wort, and yellow dock root would be excellent to improve skin health. Turmeric capsules can help clear up psoriasis.

A folk remedy worth trying on either condition is to apply raw potato juice (made in a juicer) to the affected area. Look for salves to apply topically that include aloe vera, burdock, calendula, chickweed, comfrey, echinacea, gold-

Homeopathy for Improving Skin Conditions

- *Bromium* is used for acne, boils, pimples, hard glands, and pustules.
- *Hepar sulphuris calcareum* is an important remedy for skin abscesses and acne related to youth, sensitive skin, and ulcers that burn and sting. It is also employed for recurring patches of reddened skin.
- *Kali bromatum* helps clear acne with itching that is likely to be worse on the face, chest, and shoulders. The person with this condition is likely to have a flushed face.
- *Ledum palustre* is used to dispel hard tiny bumps that occur mostly on the upper arms and thighs. It is also indicated for the patient who has itchy feet and ankles.
- *Natrum muriaticum* helps eczema that is raw and red, cold sores, oily skin, warts on the palms, and dry eruptions on the elbows, scalp periphery, and behind the ears.
- *Urtica urens* is a classic remedy for allergic reactions on the skin, rashes, insect bites, and hives that sting.

enseal, plantain, Saint John's wort, green tea, and/or tea tree oil. Use only the best quality and most natural moisturizers for your skin.

Essential oils (applied topically) that best help clear up eczema and psoriasis include bergamot, Roman chamomile, geranium, jasmine, lavender, lemon, lemon balm (melissa), neroli, rose, sandalwood, or tea tree in a jojoba base. Vitamins A, C, and E and zinc may be helpful.

Always do your best to determine and correct the cause of an ailment. Illness can be a great opportunity to learn more about health.

Here are some homeopathic suggestions for eczema and psoriasis:

- ***Alumina*** is for dry skin with dry eczema. The patient might scratch till bleeding occurs. Being in a warm bed worsens the condition.
- ***Arsenicum*** helps dry, scaly skin that often flakes off into a fine powder. Scratching does not give relief but makes it worse. Use for eczema that is worsened by cold and more intense in winter.
- ***Graphites*** aids eczema that oozes a yellow liquid and that is worse in a warm bed. This can be used for eczema that occurs around the ears, eyelids, lips, anal and genital regions, and/or skin folds of the arms and legs.
- ***Petroleum*** is a remedy for eczema that occurs on the soles of the feet, palms, and fingertips.
- ***Psorinum*** is used more for people with a cold constitution.
- ***Sulfur*** is used more for people with a hot constitution.

Herbs that benefit normal skin include chamomile, dandelion leaf, and parsley. Normal skin can be enhanced with essential oils of bergamot, cedarwood, chamomile, clary sage, geranium, jasmine, lavender, neroli, nutmeg, rose, rosewood, and/or ylang-ylang.

Sensitive skin can be soothed with essential oils of chamomile, coriander, cumin, cypress, geranium, green tea, lavender, melissa (lemon balm), palmarosa, patchouli, rose, rosewood, sandalwood, spearmint, and/or vetivert. Teas to soothe sensitive skin might include chamomile, comfrey leaf, marshmallow root, red clover blossom, or green tea.

Cleansing the Skin

Cleansing helps remove the outer layer of dead skin cells, pollutants, and makeup. It is beneficial to know what your skin type is. Emotions, hormones, menstrual cycles, weather, physical changes, weight fluctuations, and, of course, stress all affect our skin type. Cleansing is ideally done morning and night. Never go to bed with a dirty face. In the morning, cleansing might be as simple as a rinse with warm water, if your skin is very dry.

Many soaps leave a film on the skin. Antibacterial soaps, like antibiotics, destroy both good and bad bacteria, making the skin more susceptible to microbial invasion and fungal overgrowth. Bar soaps can be overly drying to the face. Transparent, or glycerin, soaps are the least drying but can contain ingredients that clog the pores. Deodorant soaps are usually irritating and chemical laden. Acne soaps can contain irritating ingredients. Superfatted soaps have extra oils but often contain beeswax and petroleum by-products, which can clog pores and cause breakouts. "Castile soap" is a term used to describe a very mild soap that usually is made with coconut, olive, or hemp seed oil, though it can still contain sodium hydroxide, which can be irritating to the skin.

The average person might only use soap under the arms, between the legs, and perhaps on the chest and back if the skin is oily. It is best to not use soap from the neck up. Soap cleans so thoroughly that it can strip and irritate the skin.

Acid and alkaline pH levels (pH stands for "potential of hydrogen") range from 0.0 (totally acid) to 14.0 (totally alkaline); 7.0 is considered neutral. If you do use soap, look for one with a low pH, between 5 and 6. Though the skin has a pH of 4.5 to 5.5, a slightly alkaline solution is more cleansing. Many bar soaps have a pH between 9 and 10. If you have oily skin or acne, a slightly higher pH is desirable. Soaps with a pH of 7 or higher can dissolve keratin and protein, might irritate dry and sensitive skin, and can increase the presence of bacteria. A mild facial cleanser is more ideal than soap, especially for mature skin.

These days there are many wonderful natural cosmetics available at natural food stores. There is something delightful about making what is good for your skin type, not to mention the lovely art of taking time to do nurturing things for yourself that are kind to the Earth Mother. Make small batches and see what benefits you.

Water for Beauty

Water symbolizes deep inner awareness, flowing movement, intuition, and subtle power. It is most symbolic of the origin of life. According to *The Urantia Book* (Urantia Foundation, 1999), life was planted in the ocean in three different places.

Water is a highly efficient conductor of energy, transmitting electrical and magnetic currents with a minimum of resistance. It absorbs, communicates, and is a universal solvent. Natural waters, such as hot springs and oceans, carry a superior vibrational pattern. Soaking in these waters fosters healing, cleansing, and rejuvenation.

Water is a universal remedy. It is abundant, available, economical, safe, and easy to use. There are millions of nerve endings in the skin that transfer hydrotherapy's healing properties.

The chlorine in many city water supplies helps destroy harmful microbes, but it can compromise the skin's acid mantle, making the skin and scalp drier and more susceptible to irritation. Chlorine is absorbed through our pores and goes right into our bloodstream. The heated water in showers produces chloroform, which, when inhaled, can make us more prone to allergies, respiratory disorders, and under-eye puffiness.

continued

Using Skin Cleansers

Moisten your skin with hot water before applying cleanser. Cleanse for a full minute to dislodge oil and dirt. Avoid scrubbing; use gentle action. Rinse well, using about thirty splashes of warm water and ending with a splash of cool water. Pat the skin dry, leaving a damp film on the skin. If your face feels tight after cleaning, it may be due to not having rinsed enough.

Whenever your face needs to be wiped, as with makeup removal, avoid using synthetic cotton balls or paper tissues, which contain irritating particles that can scratch the skin. When removing makeup from the delicate eye area, use a natural cotton ball moistened with almond oil. If you use a washcloth, it is best to use it one time only and then wash it, as washcloths can harbor bacteria by remaining moist. Cleanse your face morning and night, and never go to bed with makeup on your face.

Soft water (rainwater) dissolves easily with soap, and hard water is rich in minerals (such as calcium and magnesium) and less easy to dissolve. With hard water it can take twice as much cleanser, soap, or shampoo to achieve the same level of cleanliness that can be achieved with soft water. Hard water also combines with the mineral ions in the water and forms a film that does not completely rinse off. This same film can clog pores and coat the hair. Install a shower filter or a water filter for the entire home to safeguard your health and leave your skin and hair more radiant.

Some city water systems use ultraviolet light to kill bacteria, which reduces the need for chemicals. Water softening companies use an ion exchange system that uses sodium as a softening agent. Chemical water softeners change water's chemical makeup, and the appliances that contain them have high salt levels, which can contribute to high blood pressure.

Lemon Yogurt Cleanser

This cleanser is great for oily and acne-prone skin.

- 4 tablespoons freshly squeezed lemon juice
- 4 tablespoons plain yogurt

Combine the lemon juice and yogurt, and store in a jar in the refrigerator. Apply to face and neck, and gently remove with a piece of natural cotton.

Acne Cleanser

This can clear up stubborn breakouts. Use it as a cleanser for your entire face, or just on problem areas.

- 1/4 cup distilled witch hazel
- 20 drops lavender essential oil

Combine the witch hazel and essential oil in a clean glass jar and shake. Apply to problem areas with a cotton ball.

Foaming Cleanser

So simple! Use lemon juice for combination skin, yogurt for dry skin, or apple cider vinegar for oily skin. Because this cleanser is also a scrub, limit its use to a few times per week.

- 1 tablespoon baking soda
- 1 teaspoon freshly squeezed lemon juice, yogurt, or apple cider vinegar

Combine the ingredients in a small bowl. Wet face and gently massage into skin. Rinse well with lukewarm water.

Dry Skin Cleansing Oil

Your skin will thank you for this rich, fragrant blend.

2 tablespoons pure raw coconut or jojoba oil
18 drops jasmine or rose essential oil

Put the ingredients into an amber bottle and shake well. To use, apply some of the mixture to your face, and remove with a natural cotton ball.

Cleansing Grains

It's easy to make your own cleansing grains. This can be used up to twice a week. Store the grains in a glass jar in the bathroom. (Also see the section on scrubs, pages 41–44.)

2 cups white clay
1 cup ground rolled oats
1/4 cup ground almonds
1–2 drops lavender or geranium essential oil

Combine all the ingredients in a large bowl. Put a quarter-size portion in the palm of your hand, moisten with a bit of water, and apply to your face. Use in gentle circular movements over your skin. Rinse well.

Natural Cleansers

You can also use blended fruit as a natural cleanser. When preparing fruit for breakfast or a snack, save a bit to use for this beauty ritual. Blend one to two teaspoons of fresh fruit (preferably organic) with enough tepid water to make a purée. Apply this mixture to your face, though you can include other parts of your body. Leave it on for one minute while massaging it into your skin; then rinse it off. If you use fruits that have been chemically treated, avoid using the peels.

The best choices for fresh fruit cleansers are apricots, avocados, cantaloupe, cucumbers, green or red grapes (not purple), papayas, strawberries, and tomatoes. Other substances that can be used for cleansing include honey, olive oil, potatoes (great for blemished skin), beets, string beans, yogurt, wine, and the foam from beer. *continued*

Facial Steams

A facial steam is an excellent way to do a deep cleansing, relax muscles, and improve circulation as you give yourself an invigorating, rosy glow.

Wash your face first. Pour one quart of boiling water over a handful of herbs or seven drops of essential oil in a heatproof glass bowl. Tie your hair back. Drape a towel over your head to create a tent over the steaming bowl and your face. Keep your face about ten inches away from the water source to avoid getting burned as you inhale the sensuous steam for five to seven minutes.

Facial steams can be done once or twice a month, or before special occasions when you want to look your most radiant. Those with badly blemished skin should avoid steaming, as it can activate oil glands. Those with broken facial capillaries should also avoid steams, as they can cause increased skin redness.

Herbs for Facial Steams

Select the appropriate herbs for your skin type. Facial steams can be followed with a facial scrub and then a mask.

- **Acne:** lavender, red clover blossoms, or strawberry leaves.
- **Blackheads:** elder flowers or rosemary.
- **Combination Skin:** chamomile, lavender, licorice, or peppermint.
- **Dry Skin:** chamomile, comfrey leaves, elder flowers, fennel seed, lavender, licorice, red clover, or roses.
- **Oily Skin:** eucalyptus leaves, juniper berries, lavender, lemongrass, lemon peel, peppermint, pine, sage, or strawberry leaves.
- **Sensitive Skin:** calendula or chamomile.

For oily skin, a cleanser could be made of yogurt mixed with sea salt. Sea vegetables can be used, as they are cleansing, stimulating, detoxifying, and tonifying. Soak any type of powdered sea vegetable in tepid water for twenty minutes before using. Spread the mixture over your face and gently massage. Rolled oats or cornmeal can be powdered and mixed with milk, yogurt, or water and used as a very gentle cleanser. Baking soda can be used as an exfoliant and anti-inflammatory agent. Granulated sugar can be used as a natural exfoliant. Even though we should do our best to avoid eating sugar, it is quick dissolving and helps to cleanse and clear the skin. First cleanse your skin; then apply a light coating of coconut oil. Use about one teaspoon of sugar and apply it to several spots on your face. Use small circular motions, being careful not to stretch your skin.

Masks

Masks are beneficial for many reasons: they thoroughly cleanse the skin, increase blood circulation to the skin, improve muscle tone, soften and improve the skin's texture, and can help prevent wrinkles, lines, and other signs of aging. They can also provide a psychological lift and healthy-looking glow, thus helping you put your best face forward before special events.

There are three basic types of facial masks: detoxifying masks are for deep cleansing and help draw impurities out of the skin; hydrating masks are for deep moisturizing and are especially beneficial for dry skin; toning masks tighten and firm, which is especially beneficial for aging skin that is lacking elasticity. We don't really know the long-term effects of chemical peel-off masks. Some estheticians speculate that overuse can thin the protective stratum corneum layer.

Masks may be done once or twice a week and are always applied to cleansed skin. Avoid fruit masks if the skin is sunburned, windburned, or overly irritated. Avoid applying masks to the delicate area around the eyes. If you are allergic to something internally, do not apply it to your skin. Skin types that should avoid exfoliating agents altogether include those with eczema, rosacea, dermatitis, or seborrhea, unless recommended by a competent health professional. If a mask becomes uncomfortable or itchy, rinse it off right away.

There are many types of masks that can be made in your kitchen from fresh ingredients that can be used to nourish the skin. These are fun to use, cost effective, and free of preservatives. Simply mash the ingredients in a bowl with a fork, or process them in a blender or food processor, if necessary. You may even use the pulp from your juicer to make a facial mask, if you've just juiced something appropriate (see the list on page 35). You can also simply rub a slice of raw fruit or vegetable over your skin (face, neck, arms, the back of your hands, or any other area that is frequently exposed). My favorites include apple, cucumber, melon, potato, peach, tomato, or the inside of an avocado skin.

Apply the mask to your face and let it work while you relax for about ten to twenty minutes in the bathtub, lie on a slant board, give yourself a pedicure, or meditate.

Scrubbing is one way to exfoliate the skin. Another way is through the use of products that contain alpha hydroxy acids (AHAs). With their natural chemicals, these products exfoliate the skin without scrubbing. Fruit, yogurt, sugar, milk, buttermilk, and wine all contain the much touted alpha hydroxy acids, which stimulate new cell growth, reduce pore size, minimize fine lines, promote the retention of moisture, and result in younger-looking skin. AHAs help loosen the bond between dead skin and the living layers beneath, leaving us with a youthful glow as healthier cells come to the surface. AHAs are often found in cleansers, toners, moisturizers, and even in some makeups. It is best if they appear second or third on an ingredient list. This makes it more likely that the product contains 5 percent or more AHAs. Anything less than 1 percent is ineffective. Amounts higher than 8–15 percent are more likely to cause skin irritation. The effects of AHAs have not been studied over the long term. If AHAs are chemical derived or are overused, they might damage DNA and be a contributing factor in skin cancer due to increased sun exposure. AHAs are best for sun-damaged, thickened, and dry skin. Alpha hydroxy acids are found in grapefruits, lemons, limes, and oranges, and to a lesser degree in strawberries, blackberries, apples, tomatoes, grapes, peaches, and kiwis. Avoid using citrus fruits on dry skin.

Natural Ingredients for Homemade Masks

Many common foods can be used to make excellent, fresh, beautifying masks. If a mask needs to be thickened, add a bit of powdered rolled oats or cosmetic clay as a thickening agent. For dry skin, the addition of some oil to a fruit mask can decrease its drying potential. If the mask needs to be moistened, use a floral water (such as rose or orange flower water), honey, or yogurt. Leave the mask on for about twenty minutes. Rinse the mask off, splash with cool water, pat dry with a towel, finish with a toner, then apply a moisturizer. After a mask, it is good to moisturize twice, as masks can draw out toxins as well as moisture. Be your most beautiful self! (If you are allergic to any of the following ingredients as a food, do not use them on your skin.)

- **Almonds** can be ground and mixed with water. Almonds make a good mask for dry, mature skin, blackheads, and enlarged pores. Almonds are emollient and cleansing when shelled and finely ground. Their effect is calming and lubricating.
- **Apple purée** benefits dry, mature, oily, sensitive, and blemished skin. Apple is exfoliating, mildly antiseptic, astringent, and soothing.
- **Apricots** enliven tired, dry, normal, or oily skin and prevent wrinkles. Apricots promote cellular regeneration.
- **Avocados** are highly nutritive and softening. They contain penetrating oils for very dry, sensitive, normal, and mature skin.
- **Bananas** are nourishing for sensitive, dry, normal, and mature skin. Banana pulp helps the skin stay soft and free of impurities.
- **Barley meal** is specific for acne, oily, and sensitive skin.
- **Brewer's yeast** and **nutritional yeast** are nourishing, deeply cleansing, and good for mature and oily skin. They have a tightening effect and enliven dull-looking skin.
- **Cabbage** masks help resolve blemished, oily, and combination skin.
- **Carrot** pulp, left from making juice, helps nourish the skin and treat blemishes. It is antiseptic and good for all skin types.
- **Cherries** can be used as a facial for dry skin.
- **Clay** absorbs toxins, clears the skin, improves circulation, and is cleansing and anti-inflammatory. Clay masks can even be applied to the thighs and upper arms after weight loss to help tighten and tonify tissue. (See Resources, page 229, for specifics on the various types of clay available.)
- **Cucumbers** are cooling, astringent, and soothing for oily skin, combination skin, enlarged pores, and sensitive skin. Cucumbers also make a cooling mask when we feel overheated. Cucumber lightens freckles, calms sunburn, and helps reduce puffiness and inflammation.
- **Grapes** are cooling and soothing and help lighten and smooth uneven pigmentation. Grapes clean out imbedded oils and dirt and can be used for dry, normal, or oily skin. Grapes help heal chapped skin.
- **Green leafy herbs** like dandelion leaf, malva, and violet can be puréed in the blender and applied as detoxifying and nourishing facial masks.
- **Honey** moisturizes and tightens. It is very nutritive, softening, and lifting. Honey is an antibacterial agent. It is good for lackluster skin, enlarged pores, dry and sensitive skin, and blackheads. Honey is naturally acid balanced. Apply honey on your face and neck, then gently tap over the area for two minutes. Rinse well.
- **Kale** tonifies and rejuvenates the skin.

- **Kiwifruit** contains alpha hydroxy acids and vitamin C. It helps soften the skin and dissolve dead skin cells.
- **Lemon** lightens uneven pigment and liver spots. It is antiseptic and helps restore normal acid balance to the skin. Lemon tightens enlarged pores, is astringent and tonifying, and is best for combination and oily skin. Dilute with equal parts water before using.
- **Lettuce** is used as a mask for sensitive and oily skin.
- **Melons** soothe, tonify, and lighten the skin. They are specific for normal and oily skin.
- **Mint leaves** are ideal for acne, blemished skin, and enlarged pores. Mint is antiseptic, anti-inflammatory, cleansing, nourishing, and improves circulation.
- **Oats (powdered rolled oats)** make an excellent mask for acne, blackheads, dry or oily skin, and wrinkles.
- **Papaya** is exfoliating and helps get rid of dead skin cells. Papaya benefits oily and dry skin. Unripe green papaya is even more effective, as it contains more enzymes. You can buy green papaya powder that is processed at a low temperature (see Resources, page 229).
- **Parsley** as a mask calms blackheads, blotchy skin, and troubled complexions. Parsley tonifies and rejuvenates the skin.
- **Peaches** enliven tired, irritated, normal, and dry skin. They are anti-inflammatory and prevent wrinkles.
- **Pears** can be used as a mask for dry, normal, combination, and oily skin. They calm sore, inflamed, blotchy skin and sunburn.
- **Persimmons** make a suitable mask for all skin types.
- **Pineapple** is rich in enzymes and rejuvenating. Use it as a facial mask for dull skin tone.
- **Potatoes** make an excellent mask for acne, dry, oily, and normal skin and can calm sunburn.
- **Pumpkins** contain enzymes that exfoliate the skin and have anti-inflammatory properties.
- **Sea vegetables** are used as a mask for dehydrated skin and can firm loose, sagging, and mature skin. Sea vegetables tonify, stimulate, detoxify, refresh, and cleanse. They also soothe sun-damaged skin.
- **Strawberries** are especially good for cleansing and tightening the pores and lightening uneven skin pigmentation. Use for oily and combination skin and for calming blemishes. They help eliminate dead skin cells and feel cool and refreshing when we're overheated.

- **Tomatoes** refine pores, help eliminate blackheads, and exfoliate. Tomatoes are good for dry, blemished, sensitive, acne-prone, and oily skin. They help to restore the natural acid balance of the skin and lighten skin discolorations.
- **Turmeric** can be mixed with powdered rolled oats and yogurt. In Asian medicine, turmeric is used to promote a softer, lighter, and healthier complexion.
- **Watercress** makes a good facial for oily skin and is very refreshing.
- **Watermelon** is refreshing and astringent. It is good for dry and oily skin.
- **Yogurt** lightens uneven pigmentation. Use plain yogurt as a mask for oily, mature, or blemished skin, or for large pores. It kills harmful bacteria that makes skin blemish-prone.

Fruit Mask

Nourishing and invigorating!

3 tablespoons fresh fruit (such as apricot, pear, or peach)
3 teaspoons honey (optional)
1 teaspoon plain yogurt or water, if needed

Mash the fruit with a fork and stir in the honey. Add the yogurt if the mixture is too thick. Apply to your face and neck. Lie down (on a slant board, if you have one) for 20 minutes and relax. Rinse well.

Acne Drying Mask

This can be applied to problem areas only.

2 tablespoons powdered rolled oats or clay
2 tablespoons freshly squeezed lemon juice or apple cider vinegar

Mix into a paste and apply to pimples and bumps. Allow it to dry before rinsing off.

Moisturizing the Skin

Drinking more water is the key to moist skin. Each of our skin cells contains about 95 percent water. Moisturizers add and help our skin retain moisture by sealing in the moisture already in our skin. They also "plump" the skin, making fine lines less visible.

After every time you cleanse your skin, a moisturizer should be applied, as water helps to keep the skin's outer layers from drying out and oil seals it in. It is best to apply moisturizer to damp skin to help seal in liquid. Even oily complexions need some moistening around the eye and mouth area, which are the first to show signs of aging. Using a light moisturizer, even on oily skin, can help calm the skin and may actually encourage less oil production by providing what is needed. For normal to oily skin, a moisturizing lotion is usually more appropriate. For dry skin, look for a moisturizing cream.

A good moisturizer will be emollient and provide the skin with lubrication. Humectants attract water to the skin and are another important constituent of moisturizers. Anti-irritants might be another component and are beneficial whether the irritation comes from the sun, pollution, or skin care products. Comfrey leaf and root, aloe vera, licorice root, marshmallow root, chamomile flower, white willow bark, and vitamin C are all considered anti-irritants. Coconut oil, cocoa butter, and extra-virgin olive oil or any raw oil are emollient and can help create a thin, imperceptible layer that re-creates the soothing benefits that our own skin produces and prevents moisture evaporation.

Phospholipids act as humectants and prevent water evaporation. They are the only known substance that can form liposomes, which carry nourishment to the skin and even create moisture reservoirs within the skin. Antioxidants in a moisturizer can reduce or prevent some of the free radical damage our skin is exposed to. Antioxidants include alpha lipoic acid, green tea, beta-carotene, vitamins C and E, selenium, zinc, beta-glucan, and coenzyme Q10.

Avoid poor-quality cosmetics that contain mineral oil, chemicals, and/or artificial colors and fragrances. Products that have beeswax as the main ingredient may be too heavy and waxy for anything other than extremely dry skin. Use the lightest moisturizer that makes your skin feel soft without feeling oily. Some skin types might benefit from using moisturizers only on dry spots.

Use upward circular movements or small tapping movements until the moisturizer is rubbed in. Alternatively, wait about ten minutes for the moisturizer to be absorbed into the skin, then gently massage in any remainder. Start at the outward corner of your eye and move inward toward your nose, then continue in a circle around your eyelid, returning to the starting position. When touching the eye area to moisturize, the best way is to gently press the skin, rolling your finger gently and working from the inner corner of the eye out. Do not force the skin to be moved, as this can weaken collagen. Dab moisturizer. Be sure to moisturize the eye area at least twice daily. Always use love and care when touching your skin. Avoid using tissues or synthetic cotton balls, which can cause tiny scratches or splinters. If you use cotton, make sure it is the real thing.

Clothing protects most of our anatomy, but our facial skin is almost always exposed to the elements. Remember to moisturize not only the face but the neck, chest, hands, and feet.

Those with dry skin should moisturize even at a young age. Those over age thirty-five should use a body moisturizer. Moisturize morning, noon, and night. After moisturizing, you can spritz your face with an aromatherapy facial spray.

Combine 1/2 cup distilled water with 1 teaspoon of vodka and 1/4 teaspoon essential oil in a clean spray bottle. Shake well and mist your face with your eyes and mouth closed.

To apply facial oils, mix 15 drops of essential oil to 1 ounce carrier oil. Apply after cleansing your face. Lie down and relax for ten minutes. Tissue off any excess.

My favorite oil for moisturizing is coconut, as it is available raw and smells delightful. Olive oil is also available cold pressed. Here are some other classic carrier oils for lubricating the body:

- **Dry Skin:** almond, avocado, olive, black sesame, sesame, or walnut oils.
- **Oily Skin:** almond, apricot kernel, or grapeseed oil.
- **Sensitive Skin:** almond, apricot kernel, coconut, olive, or sunflower oils.

Serums

Serums are lightweight, gel-like moisturizers that are less oily or emollient than a moisturizer and are often infused with antioxidants. They are usually applied under moisturizer, or alone at night, as a way to deeply nourish the skin. Are they absolutely necessary? No, but they can be beneficial.

In general, to make your own moisturizer, use room-temperature ingredients and one part oil to one part water. To keep the mixture from separating, always put the oil in the blender first and gradually add water.

Simple Scented Moisturizer

This is delicious, but don't eat it; put it on your skin!

2 tablespoons softened coconut oil
5 drops essential oil of your choice

Allow the coconut oil to get to room temperature, and mash in the essential oil with a fork. Rub into your skin.

Herbal Oil

This is a basic preparation in any Herbology 101 class that even Harry Potter learned.

1 cup carrier oil (such as olive, almond, or coconut)
1/2 cup dried herbs of your choice

Crush the herbs with a mortar and pestle. Add to the oil and place in a clean, dry glass jar and stir well. Allow to steep for two weeks. Strain (the herbs may be composted) and keep the oil.

Mindy's Moisturizer

Mindy Green is one of North America's foremost herbalists and aromatherapists (and one of my best friends). This moisturizer can be used on the face and body.

3/4 ounce beeswax

1 cup vegetable oil (such as almond)

1 cup water

30–50 drops essential oil of your choice

Grate the beeswax, add the oil, and gently heat in a double boiler. When the wax has melted, allow it to cool for a few minutes, but not long enough for it to harden. Place the lid on a blender and remove the center plug. Using a wide-mouth funnel (to reduce splattering), pour the water into the blender. Turn the blender on at high speed while slowly adding the oil and wax mixture. When about three-quarters of the oil has been added, the mixture will begin to harden. Turn the blender off and stir. Restart the blender and add the rest of the oil mixture. Then add the essential oils. Don't overblend. Put the moisturizer into clean wide-mouth containers. Store any extra in the refrigerator.

Dry Brush Skin Massage

Brushing our skin is as important as brushing our hair and teeth, and should be done daily. It wakes up the body, removes dead layers of skin, helps keep pores unclogged, improves blood and lymphatic circulation, stimulates the nerve endings, strengthens the immune system, decreases cellulite, rejuvenates the complexion, and promotes a youthful radiance. That's a lot of benefits!

Buy a soft vegetable fiber brush designed for this purpose at your natural food store. Many are made of boar bristle, but palm fibers are a vegan alternative, and have a long detachable wooden handle, which makes it easy to reach all body parts. Check the bristles by rubbing them on your palm to make sure they are not too scratchy. If the bristles are too stiff, you can moisten them or you can get a softer brush. Avoid using synthetic bristles, as they are too sharp and can damage the skin. Each family member should have his or her own brush.

Avoid brushing areas of the skin that are irritated or infected. Brush your skin when it is dry, before bathing. Disrobe, and begin gently brushing the skin in small circles or in one direction upward toward the heart, focusing on areas of about eight to ten inches. Starting with your feet and between your toes, work from the feet to the ankles, ankles to the knees, and knees to the thighs, upper thighs, then buttocks. Continue on to the hands and between the fingers; then move to the wrists and elbows, and from the elbows to the underarms and shoulders. Brush your stomach, chest, back, and neck. Of course, be gentle over the face, inner thighs, and breasts; you can avoid the genitals. The massage should feel pleasurable, not painful. Afterward, shower or bathe. You can end with cool water to give yourself an invigorating circulatory massage. Every two weeks, wash your skin brush and dry it in the sun or a warm place.

Scrubs

Scrubs help remove dead skin cells from the skin's surface. The epidermis is constantly shedding, about a layer a day, and there are about thirty layers. As skin ages, the cellular renewal decreases somewhat, and if dead cells are not removed, the skin will look dull. Scrubs can help unblock and loosen oily plugs that fill the pores. They help remove dead skin cells, distribute oils, improve circulation, and stimulate cell renewal. Epidermabrasion, or exfoliation, means massaging with light friction, or sloughing off the skin. Scrubs can help beautify dry, aging, flaky, oily, rough-textured, and blackhead- and acne-prone skin. Exfoliating is an important process for women over thirty-five to promote a youthful complexion. Men are less likely to get facial lines, partially because they do a frequent epidermabrasion by shaving.

Overusing exfoliants, including cleansing grains and scrubs, can aggravate and age sensitive skin by making it more susceptible to sun damage, destroying the hydrolipid barrier, changing the pH of the acid mantle, and exposing the skin to chemicals (when chemical-based products are used). Scrubs are not recommended in cases of severe acne, spider veins, or very sensitive skin, as scrubs can cause irritation. Use caution, as scrubbing too harshly can tear the skin, and abrasive scrubs can literally cut the skin. Treat blemished skin very gently. Avoid scrubbing moles, warts, and varicose veins. Excess scrubbing can result in broken capillaries. People with skin problems caused by illness or disease should avoid scrubs or proceed carefully with any exfoliation until they can find other ways to clear up their skin problem.

Most facial scrubs are made of dried ingredients that are moistened before being applied to the skin. Tie your hair back when doing a scrub or mask. If your skin is delicate, dilute the scrub with water; you can eventually use less water as the skin gradually becomes used to being scrubbed. The most abrasive effect of a scrub will occur when it is applied to dry skin. You can scrub using a complexion brush or your fingers. Rolled oats or cornmeal can be powdered in a blender and mixed with milk, yogurt, or water and used as a very gentle cleanser. The best scrubs for skin prone to breakouts include finely powdered oats, barley, or rice. Avoid commercial scrubs that contain waxy ingredients; they actually clog the pores. Scrubs should rinse off easily.

You can also exfoliate other areas of the body where dead skin accumulates, such as the feet, elbows, and knees. Loofahs, which are made from the skeleton of a gourd, are absorbent, to some degree, and become flexible when wet. Loofahs are rougher than a sponge and make an excellent exfoliating agent; they are best used with circular strokes. Loofahs should always be used wet so they don't scratch the skin, but they tend to be too irritating for areas from the neck up. They are convenient for using with cleansing ingredients. As a loofah has an open structure that allows air to pass through it, it is less likely to collect bacteria than a sponge or washcloth. After each use, rinse it and hang it up to dry to prevent mold and mildew from forming. Alternatively, dry it in the sun between uses. You can also put your loofah in the dishwasher or washing machine every couple of weeks.

A *tawashi* is a Japanese scrubbing brush. It is good for most of the body, but not the face, and should be used only gently over the breasts, inner arms, and inner thighs. An ayate cloth is made of the desert agave plant and woven into a loose cloth that can be used as an exfoliator. Facial brushes and washcloths are scrubbing tools, but they are hard to keep clean and harbor bacteria. They also tend to exfoliate only the very surface of the skin. Be sure to regularly cleanse any scrubbing tools.

Body scrubs eliminate outer layers of dead skin and leave you refreshed. They are great after bodywork and when you want to feel extra smooth and invigorated. A body scrub should be done while standing in a dry tub, to avoid making a mess. First take a brief shower to remove excess dirt. Dip a washcloth into a scrub mixture and, using a circular motion, massage it into your skin. Be sure to avoid any cuts or wounds. Keep dipping into the scrub mixture until your entire body has been scrubbed and the solution is gone. Be gentle. Rinse with warm water; do not use soap.

To do a salt scrub, shower first. Then massage olive oil into your skin. Next, moisten salt with lemon juice and massage it into your skin. Use a loofah or washcloth to gently rub in the salt until you feel a glowing, warm sensation. Shower to remove the salt.

Scrubs can be moistened with water, milk, yogurt, buttermilk, honey, wine, or fresh fruit juice. The following are a few of the many common ingredients that can be used in scrubs.

- **Almonds,** when ground, are an effective cleanser for sensitive, dry skin. However, if you scrub too harshly, they can cause tiny tears in the skin.
- **Baking soda** makes a very simple scrub that is not overly abrasive.
- **Barley powder** is soothing, softening, and useful for all skin types, though it is ideal for dry, mature, or sensitive skin. Barley powder can be made by grinding 1/2 cup whole barley in the blender.
- **Cornmeal** can be used as a scrub. The larger grains are more abrasive than finer cornmeal.

- **Kelp** is rich in minerals and ideal for mature skin. Those with very sensitive skin can sometimes find sea vegetables irritating.
- **Oats (powdered rolled oats)** soothe, absorb oil, cleanse, and soften the skin. Oats are ideal for acne and dry, mature, or sensitive skin.
- **Rice** that has been finely powdered in a blender gives the skin a polished appearance. It is a favorite in Asia.
- **Sea salt** makes an ideal scrub to soften the skin. Salt sloughs off dead skin cells, invigorates the skin, and increases circulation. Sometimes referred to as "salt glows," salt stimulates the skin, muscles, and nerves and improves the texture of tired, bumpy, and dull skin. Salt can sting on an open cut, so avoid putting it on open wounds. Salt scrubs are somewhat abrasive and best used for exfoliation, stimulation, and cleansing. Salt can be drying if not used with something emollient, such as coconut oil. Avoid salt scrubs on the face or on dry, damaged, or delicate skin.
- **Sesame seeds** can be finely ground and used for cleansing dry or sensitive skin.
- **Sugar** contains glycolic acid. It stimulates, lightens, moisturizes, and wakes up dry, sagging skin.

Sugar Herb Scrub

Don't eat sugar. Instead, use it as a good exfoliating ingredient; it contains minerals in its raw form.

1 cup raw sugar

1/4 cup powdered lavender flowers

Combine the ingredients and store in a clean wide-mouth jar. To use, place a small amount into your palm, add a bit of water, and massage into your face, thighs, buttocks, feet, and hands. Rinse well.

Salt Scrub

This scrub is alkalinizing.

1/4 cup sea salt

5 drops lavender essential oil

1/4 cup olive or almond oil

Place the salt in a bowl, and stir in the essential oil and olive oil. To use, place a small amount into your palm, add a bit of water, and massage into your face, thighs, buttocks, feet, and hands. Rinse well. Makes one treatment.

Simple Scrub

Here's a macrobiotic version.

- 1/2 cup powdered rolled oats
- 1/4 cup fine cornmeal

Combine the ingredients and store in a clean wide-mouth jar. To use, place a small amount into your palm, add a bit of water, and massage into your face, thighs, buttocks, feet, and hands. Rinse well.

Oatmeal Corn Almond Scrub

Here's another simple variation.

- 3 tablespoons powdered rolled oats
- 3 tablespoons cornmeal
- 3 tablespoons ground almonds
- 1 tablespoon honey

Combine all the ingredients in a bowl and store in a glass jar with a lid. Put some of the mixture into your hands and add a bit of water or yogurt to moisten. Use small circular massage strokes on your skin for two minutes. Rinse well.

Cleansing Grains

Try this with your favorite essential oils.

- 1 cup ground oats
- 1/4 cup ground almonds
- 1–2 drops lavender or geranium essential oil

Combine the ingredients in a bowl. Store in a glass jar.

Toners

Toners are often referred to as fresheners, clarifiers, tonics, or astringents. However, astringents tend to include more alcohol than a toner. Toners are nourishing and tonifying and are often antiseptic and astringent. Toners are best applied after cleansing the skin but before moisturizing or applying makeup. They feel fresh and energizing, brighten a mood, and can even calm a hot flash. In a pinch, you can use your toner as a cleanser.

The skin contains a protective acid mantle composed of mature skin cells, bacteria, sweat, and sebum. The skin's naturally low pH protects it from infection, including acne and boils. Chemical skin products can easily damage the acid mantle. Most soaps are overly alkaline and can damage the skin's protective acid mantle, causing it to become moisture depleted. As skin ages, it takes longer for the acid mantle to return to its normal slightly acidic state. The skin's pH is usually restored within about twenty minutes after washing, but constant exposure to synthetic creams and excessive hot bathing with chemical substances decrease this acid mantle, allowing germs to be more active. The acid mantle of the skin is ideally between pH 4.8 and 6. When the pH of a substance is lower than 7, it is considered acidic; higher than 7 is considered alkaline. Most synthetic soaps are very alkaline. Many toners contain alcohol, which can decrease oiliness and tighten pores, but can also strip the skin's natural oils and cause a leathery look. Toners containing alcohol should be used only by those with very oily skin, and make sure the alcohol content is less than 35 percent. Toners usually have less alcohol than astringents, if any.

Water-based toners may include aloe vera or vegetable glycerin; they are less astringent and more moisturizing. Floral waters can also be used as toners. Rose, chamomile, and orange flower waters nourish and moisturize dry skin. Orange, linden, and rosemary floral waters can be used for normal skin. Rosemary floral water can be used for oily skin. Lavender floral water is suitable for all skin types. Chamomile floral water is anti-inflammatory. Witch hazel can also be used as a toner for oily or acne-prone skin.

A toner is not a necessity for everyone. It is rare that a person over age thirty-five needs an astringent. If you do use a toner, you may want to use it in the morning to remove any oil that may have accumulated overnight. Use toners before serums, moisturizers, and any makeup you might use.

Apply toners with gentle upward strokes using 100-percent-cotton balls or your fingers. For more stimulation, gently tap over the face with your fingers while applying the toner. You can bottle homemade toners in clean (never used for chemicals) spray bottles. Hold the bottle about six inches from your face and spray.

Body splashes are like toners for the whole body. When misted onto the skin, they are refreshing; they also can be deodorizing and nourishing to the skin. You can also pour a bit of body splash into the palm of your hand and apply it as a pick-me-up; this is especially effective when applied to the head and neck.

A simple and easy way to tone the skin is to rub an ice cube over your face after cleansing and before moisturizing. Put two trays of ice cubes into a sink filled with cold water. While wearing rubber gloves lined with cotton, splash your face about forty times, covering all areas. Because I live in Colorado, my favorite toner is to go out on my balcony in the winter and pat on some freshly fallen snow. I visualize taking in the crystalline beauty of radiant snowflakes. Another simple way to tone the skin is to rub fruit peels over your face after eating the fruit. Use apricot or peach for dry skin; grape, lemon, or grapefruit peel for oily skin; pear for sensitive skin; and apple for blemished skin.

You can make a simple aromatherapy toner by adding 4 drops of pure essential oil to an 8-ounce spray bottle filled with mineral water, or to a mixture of 1/2 cup aloe vera juice and 1/2 cup water. Add 1 teaspoon of freshly squeezed lemon juice or 1/2 teaspoon apple cider vinegar to make the mixture more astringent for oily skin. For dry to normal skin, 1/2 teaspoon apple cider vinegar and 1/4 teaspoon oil can be added to make the mixture both tonifying and lubricating.

Simple Toner

This toner is best for oily skin.

1/2 cup witch hazel or water
1/2 cup aloe vera juice

Combine the ingredients in a clean spray bottle.

pH Balancing Toner

This helps restore normal acidity to the skin.

1 tablespoon apple cider vinegar or freshly squeezed lemon juice
1/3 cup water

Combine the ingredients in a clean spray bottle.

Rosemary Toner

This feels invigorating to your skin and mind. It is suitable for all skin types.

3 tablespoons dried rosemary
2 cups water
4 teaspoons brandy

Simmer the rosemary in the water for 20 minutes. Remove from the heat and let it steep another hour. Strain and add the brandy.

Floral Water

Anoint yourself! Use a spray bottle if you like.

1 tablespoon fresh herbs
1/4 cup hot water
1 drop essential oil of your choice

Place the herbs in an 8-ounce Ball jar. Pour the hot water over the herbs and cover the jar. Allow to steep 8 to 12 hours. Strain. Add the essential oil. Store in the refrigerator for up to a week.

Toner for Dry Skin

This smells like a garden in springtime.

3/4 cup distilled water
1/4 cup rose water

Combine the ingredients in a clean spray bottle.

If you want to tighten the eye area after cleansing, apply a light coating of plain yogurt.

Floral Toner for Oily Skin

It is so easy to make something beautiful and effective.

1/2 cup rose water
2 tablespoons orange flower water
2 tablespoons witch hazel
4 drops geranium essential oil

Combine all of the ingredients in a spray bottle and shake well. Mist yourself occasionally during the day, keeping your eyes and mouth closed.

Facial Spritzer

Spritz and sparkle!

1/2 cup water
1/2 cup aloe vera juice
20 drops essential oil of your choice

Combine all the ingredients in a mister bottle and spritz above your head several times daily, allowing the cool, moistening, fragrant water to fall upon your face and lift your spirits.

Body Splash

This will refresh you and wake you up. It will keep for a month when stored in the refrigerator.

1 cup apple cider vinegar
1/2 cup chopped fresh peppermint leaves
1/4 cup chopped fresh rosemary leaves
1 quart water
Juice and peel of 1 lemon

Steep the herbs in the vinegar for 2 weeks. Strain. Add the water, lemon juice, and lemon peel, and process in the blender. Strain. Pour into a spray bottle. Splash it wherever it is needed.

Queen of Hungary Water

Queen of Hungary Water has long been esteemed as a delightful topical formula for tonifying the skin, nourishing the hair, and relieving headaches; it has also been used as an aftershave, footbath, and mouthwash. It is considered invigorating and ideal for all skin types. At one time, it was even applied topically as a liniment to arthritic, gouty, and paralyzed limbs to improve circulation.

Queen of Hungary Water is believed to have originated around the mid-1300s with Elizabeth, queen of Hungary and sister to Casimir the Great, of Poland. It was rumored to so enhance the beauty of the queen that she had twenty-five marriage proposals in her elderly years, and that when she was seventy-two, the king of Poland, then age twenty-five, asked for her hand in marriage. There is also the possibility that Queen of Hungary Water was a creation of the herbal-savvy Gypsies, who pedaled this product as they traveled across Europe under the protection of the king of Hungary.

No matter what the origins of this time-tested fluid, Queen of Hungary Water is easy to make, inexpensive, and incorporates many of the herbs that are coming up in our gardens. It makes a lovely and original gift and is an excellent beauty product.

The original versions were made with aqua vitae, brandy or vodka, and rosemary as the main herb. In recent times, the formula has evolved and become embellished; it is now often made with a gentler and less drying vinegar.

continued

Apple Cider Vinegar Peppermint Toner

This even cools a hot flash! It is excellent for tired skin with enlarged pores.

3 tablespoons chopped fresh peppermint leaves
2 tablespoons apple cider vinegar
1 cup water

Place the peppermint in the vinegar in a jar and allow it to steep for 1 week. Strain and add the water. Store the unused portion in the refrigerator.

Sun Safety

By now everyone knows that excessive sun exposure can contribute to premature aging, wrinkles, and even skin cancer. Sunlight draws toxins out of the body, where they maintain contact with the skin and are exposed to sunlight; this combination can contribute to cancer. Sun-damaged skin causes the outer layers to become thicker and more yellowed. The underlying layers of skin then generate abnormal cell growth and hypermelanin production is increased. This abnormal cellular growth can also result in malformations in elastin, degeneration of collagen, and poor circulation to the lymphatic channels and blood. Overexposure to the sun can cause blotchiness, wrinkles, and premature aging. Excess tanning and repeated sunburns cause the skin to age. Wrinkles manifest, oils and water are lost, collagen and elastin are weakened.

Although fair-skinned people do get sunburned more easily, dark-skinned people can get burned and damage their skin by excess exposure. Tanning wasn't even considered chic until after World War II.

There are three types of ultraviolet light: UVA, UVB, and UVC. Most UVCs are filtered out by the atmosphere and are less likely to reach the earth's surface, though the breakdown of the ozone layer has reduced this protection. UVAs and UVBs both reach the earth's surface. UVBs are the most likely to burn, but the earth is bombarded with one hundred times more UVAs than

UVBs. Both UVAs and UVBs stimulate the production of free radicals, and sun damage occurs when these free radicals interact with the ultraviolet rays of the sun. UVAs attack the connective tissues in the deeper layers of skin, as well as turning it a golden color. UVA exposure can contribute to premature wrinkling and aging, as well as skin cancer. Ultraviolet light suppresses the immunity of the skin and impairs the body's ability to prevent melanomas.

There is no such thing as a safe suntan. Repeated suntanning, and especially sunburns, can increase our risk of skin cancer. Drink plenty of water. Wear a wide-brimmed hat that gives shade to the back of your neck and choose light-colored, loose-fitting clothes with long sleeves that are made of a densely woven fabric. We can get burned through flimsy clothing. Cover vulnerable areas, such as your nose and back of your neck. Avoid being out in the sun between 10:00 a.m. and 4:00 p.m. (11:00 a.m. to 3:00 p.m. during daylight saving time). We can get sunburned in the water or shade, and even on a cloudy day. Watch a movie, read, or nap during the sun's most intense part of the day. We are more likely to burn at high altitudes, as the atmosphere is thinner. For every thousand-foot increase in elevation, ultraviolet ray potency increases by 4 percent. Water, cement, sand, and even grass can reflect the sun's rays, thereby intensifying them. Snow reflects 85 percent of the sun's ultraviolet rays.

UVAs can get through glass and are a primary cause of wrinkles and skin cancers. Don't even think about using a tanning bed, sunlamp, or sun reflector.

Children have a lower tolerance for the sun than adults. Never expose babies to direct sunlight, especially those who are younger than six months old.

Substances that can increase photosensitivity and the likelihood of burning include antibiotics, antidepressants, antihistamines, artificial sweeteners, birth control pills, blood pressure medications, carbonated beverages, deodorant soaps, diuretics, essential oils applied either topically or taken internally (angelica, bergamot, carrot, fennel, grapefruit, lemon, lime, neroli, orange, and parsley), hormones, Retin-A, St. John's wort, Thorazine, tranquiliz-

Queen of Hungary Water

6 parts lemon balm

4 parts chamomile flowers

4 parts rose petals

3 parts calendula flowers

3 parts comfrey leaf

2 parts elder flowers

1 part rosemary leaf

1 part sage leaf

1 part lemon or orange peel

Apple cider vinegar or vodka, as needed

Place the herbs in a sterile glass jar. Cover with apple cider vinegar or vodka. Place a piece of waxed paper, cut several inches larger than the lid, on top of the jar, then screw on the lid. This prevents the lid from rusting. Allow the mixture to sit for 2 weeks to 1 month in a sunny window, shaking the jar daily. After 2 weeks, strain out the herbs and compost them. Bottle the remaining liquid, adding 1/2 cup rose water or orange flower water (for dry skin) or 1/2 cup witch hazel (for oily skin) for every cup of herbal vinegar. Add 2 drops geranium, lavender, or rose essential oil for added fragrance. Pour the liquid into clean, attractive bottles and label them. The finished product does not need to be refrigerated. Apply the water as a toner, after cleansing and before moisturizing.

Regardless of what you believe about its origins, Queen of Hungary Water is a safe and excellent product made from beautiful, natural ingredients that can bring health and beauty into your self-care rituals.

ers, and yarrow. Chemicals known as psoralens, which are present in limes, parsley, and parsnips, can make us more sensitive to the sun if they are handled shortly before exposure. Apply perfumes to areas that are not exposed to the sun, as some perfumes may contribute to photosensitivity.

The type of fats we eat can affect how our bodies will react to the sun. Overconsumption of refined oils, like canola, corn, safflower, and soy, can increase the risk of skin cancers. Skin cancer rates have not been improved by the use of sunscreens, by and large, because they are not applied frequently enough according to manufacturer directions. Some of the chemicals in sunscreens might be a contributing factor in skin cancers, even though they give protection against burning. If you choose to use sunscreen, here are some factors you should be aware of:

- Both sunblocks and sunscreens protect the skin from sun exposure. Sunblocks are more likely to contain zinc oxide and/or titanium dioxide and form an actual physical barrier by reflecting the sun's harmful rays away from the skin.
- Sunscreens are more likely to contain benzophenones and cinnamates, which work by absorbing and scattering the sun's rays, encouraging longer wavelengths and less harm to the skin.
- Sunblocks that have sun protection factors (SPF) listed are considered over-the-counter drugs.
- The SPF number tells you how long the product will prevent you from getting sunburn. SPF 15 means you can stay in the sun fifteen times longer without reddening than you could if you wore no sunscreen at all.
- The higher the SPF number, the greater chance the product will cause skin irritation. An SPF higher than 17 should only be used when really needed.

Select sun protection creams rich in antioxidants and low in chemicals. Most sunscreens are designed to protect against UVB, the most burning rays. There are now newer ones that also protect against UVA. Zinc oxide, titanium dioxide, and avobenzone are effective and less toxic to use. Green tea, vitamin E, and pycnogenol are naturally occurring free radical scavengers that can help protect against UVAs and UVBs. Jojoba has a natural sun protection factor of about 4. Some sunscreens contain benzophenone-3, octyl methoxycinnamate, and/or octyl-dimethyl-PABA, all of which can mimic the effects of estrogen. Many people are allergic to PABA and its derivative padimate. Look for natural sunscreens at the health food store. Green coffee beans and black walnut are two botanicals with some natural sunscreen ability. Shea butter works as a mild sunscreen and helps to hold moisture in the skin.

It is best to apply sunscreens fifteen to twenty minutes before sun exposure. This gives the product time to be absorbed. Sunscreen needs to be reapplied at least every two hours. Sunscreens can be water resistant but not waterproof. Water-resistant sunscreens should be reapplied every forty to eighty minutes. Don't use waterproof sunscreens for regular daily use if you are not going to be in the water; you'll only expose yourself to more chemicals. Apply liberally. Sunscreeens in makeup might not really offer that much sun protection. Sunscreen is best applied last (after moisturizers and makeup), because putting anything over it would dilute its effectiveness. Sunscreens are now being dissolved in lakes, and are being associated with toxic estrogenic effects on fish.

Would that you could meet the sun and the wind with more of your skin and less of your raiment. For the breath of life is in the sunlight and the hand of life is in the wind.

—KAHLIL GIBRAN, *THE PROPHET*

Prevention is the key. By all means, avoid getting sunburned. However, if it happens, here are some healing techniques to cool the fire:

- Avoid further sun exposure until your symptoms have subsided. Sunburn can continue to develop for twelve to twenty-four hours after the initial burn occurs.
- After being in the sun, take a cool shower.
- Place a cool moist towel over any areas that got too much sun, and take a rest. Do not apply ice. It can take several hours for sunburn to be apparent.
- Drink plenty of water and cool peppermint tea to cool you from the inside and help rehydrate the skin.
- Soak in a tepid bath to which one cup of apple cider vinegar, one cup of powdered dry oatmeal, one cup of baking soda, or seven drops of peppermint or lavender essential oil have been added.
- Apple cider vinegar is great for minor sunburns, but if the burn is severe or deep, it may be irritating.
- Bags of black, green, or chamomile tea can be moistened and applied to the skin. Alternatively, they can be made into a tea and added to the bathwater.
- Blend some yogurt, grated raw potato, or cucumber and apply the mixture to your skin. If you like, add two drops of lavender essential oil to the mixture.
- Apply aloe vera juice with a few drops of lavender essential oil.
- For sunburned lips, apply a compress of equal parts milk and water.

- For burns with blisters relieved by cold compresses, use homeopathic *Cantharis*. Do not break the blisters.
- For minor sunburn, use homeopathic *Cantharis* or *Urtica urens*.

Anything that can burn the skin can also burn the eyes. If you do wear sunglasses, select absorptive lenses that block ultraviolet rays (99–100 percent). Gray, green, or dark brown lenses provide good viewing as well as sun protection. Red and yellow tints can minimize haze but don't offer enough protection from sun exposure; if they have a UV coating, though, they can be adequate. Blue and black colors are dark enough to impair visibility. Pastel shades don't offer adequate protection. The lens color should be uniform, not darker or lighter in different places. "UV absorption up to 400 nm" on a label means the same as 100 percent UV absorption. The most important time to wear sunglasses is between 10:00 a.m. and 4:00 p.m., when the sun's rays are strongest.

Choose sunglasses that hug your face, with wide rims and sidepieces to shield your eyes all around. One way to test glasses is to hold them out from you at arm's length. Look through them from a distance at a straight line. If the straight edge curves, moves, distorts, or has imperfections, these are not correct. However, I do recommended getting twenty minutes a day of full-spectrum light, without wearing sunglasses, and preferably not glasses or contact lenses, to aid sleep, improve mood, and maintain hormonal balance. For sunburned eyes, apply cucumber slices or chamomile tea bags over closed eyes and lie down to rest.

Ten minutes nude in the fresh air and sunlight baths in the early morning or late afternoon can be delicious medicine for the skin!

Lips

Our mouths enable us to eat, drink, speak, kiss, and engage in many other earthly delights. The lips are exposed to many environmental factors. One of the first facial signs of aging is the loss of a full lip line.

Lips are extremely sensitive to the ramifications of sun and weather, as they have no melanin and lack the oil glands that help protect against drying. People who are prone to herpes outbreaks or cold sores need to use SPF 15 or higher sunblock on their lips, as ultraviolet light can bring on an outbreak. Fluoride toothpaste can dry lips. Alcohol-containing products, like mouthwash, can be further drying. Stop licking your lips; licking will only dry them out more, since saliva contains drying enzymes.

In Asian medicine, the outer lips are governed by the health of the intestines. Dry lips can indicate a lack of internal moisture, and cracked skin around the lip area can indicate a need for the B vitamins.

Place
Stamp
Here

THE MAIL ORDER CATALOG

PO Box 180
Summertown, TN 38483

You can exfoliate the lips by coating them lightly with a vegetable oil, and then scrubbing them with a warm, wet washcloth or soft toothbrush. Then apply moisturizer.

Look for lip products that contain shea butter, cocoa butter, coconut oil, calendula, comfrey, honey, and/or vitamin E, all of which help heal and protect the lips. Remember to moisturize the upper lip area.

Here are a few exercises for beautiful, healthy lips. Do lip exercises daily for a week, then do them three times a week.

- Curl your lips around your teeth and press your lips together.
- Practice blowing out hard.
- Make a big O shape with your mouth, without stretching, just comfortably wide. Focus on the center of your upper lip, and attempt to move it down and out to a count of ten. As it curls naturally over your teeth, breathe through your nose. Slowly relax your lip, relaxing your mouth to a count of ten. Repeat two more times.

When we are attracted to another person, our lips redden. Lipstick mimics this flush of attraction. Rub a cut strawberry or raspberry over your lips to gently color them and give you delicious kisses. You can also gently color your lips with a bit of beet juice or organic red rose petals. Alkanet root will yield a reddish color and annatto seeds will give a yellowish orange shade.

In general, a good ratio for homemade lip balm is 1 part beeswax to 2.5 parts oil. Adding a little castor oil will add a bit of sheen.

Never rub off lipstick, as this removes the protective surface cells of the lips. It is better to blot it off with a tissue.

Tinted Lip Balm

Make enough of this to give as presents to your friends.

1/8 ounce alkanet root

1 cup olive oil

1/4 cup beeswax

1 tablespoon honey

5 drops essential oil (vanilla, peppermint, or cardamom)

Simmer the alkanet root in the olive oil at a low temperature for 15 minutes, or mix them together and allow them to steep in a clean, dry glass jar for two weeks. Strain, pressing the oil out of the root with clean, dry fingers. Add the beeswax and heat or reheat gently until the beeswax is melted. Remove from the heat and add the honey and essential oil. Pour into lip balm containers. Allow to cool before sealing the containers.

Coconut Lip Balm

I like this simple recipe because it is unheated.

- 4 tablespoons coconut oil
- 4 drops spearmint essential oil
- 4 drops rose essential oil
- 4 drops cardamom essential oil

Place the coconut oil in a tightly sealed jar in a pot of hot water until the oil is liquefied. Add the essential oils, stirring well. Pour immediately into small lip balm containers.

Lip Balm

Here is another variation on lip balm that makes a smaller amount.

- $4\frac{1}{2}$ teaspoons almond oil
- $\frac{1}{2}$ teaspoon vitamin E oil
- 2 teaspoons grated beeswax
- 4 drops essential oil (such as peppermint or cardamom)

Warm the almond oil and vitamin E oil in a small saucepan over low heat. Add the beeswax and stir until it is melted. Remove from the heat and stir in the essential oil. Pour into a small container with a secure lid. Cool completely before sealing the container.

Ruby Tuesday

Use this to add a hint of red color to your homemade lip balms.

- 4 ounces cold-pressed almond oil
- 1 teaspoon alkanet root

Pour the almond oil into a glass jar and add the alkanet root. Seal with a tight-fitting lid and shake the jar daily for 10 days. Press the oil out of the alkanet root. Compost the root and retain the oil.

PROBLEM SKIN

Wrinkles and Fine Lines

Many people cherish laugh lines for the character they give their face; they may also believe that wrinkles are inevitable. As we age, the body produces less collagen and elastin, the sebaceous glands become less active, and the skin tends to get lighter in color, drier, less resilient, and more vulnerable to the ravages of wind, excess sun, and intense weather. However, there are plenty of lifestyle techniques to minimize the appearance of wrinkles.

In general, wrinkles emerge in a pattern. Vertical and horizontal lines appear on the forehead; then crow's-feet around the eyes become visible. Wrinkles begin from the nose and move down to the mouth corners. As age advances, small vertical lines can appear above the upper lip, while creases appear on the eyelids. Wrinkles can make us look more tired.

Fine lines can be due to a depletion of fluids and internal moisture in the body. Some lines on the face, such as lines around the nose and mouth, are actually creases from movement rather than wrinkles resulting from damage. Fine lines are nonpermanent and often disappear when the skin is well moisturized.

Free radicals from food and sun accumulate and break down RNA and DNA, collagen, elastin, and the lipids of cellular membranes. As we age, circulation decreases, sebaceous glands function less actively, and skin becomes drier. The fat layers under the skin get thinner, making the skin appear looser. (This is why older skin looks more transparent, and why people who are overweight have fewer wrinkles.) When skin is thinner and lighter, it is more subject to drying out, burning, and eventually wrinkling.

What causes wrinkles? In Asian medicine, wrinkles are said to be due to blocked or stagnant *chi*, also known as energy or life force. Prolonged sun exposure, wind, heat, excess cold, pollution, genetics, fat depletion, rapid weight loss, slow epidermal renewal, lack of rest and sleep, poor-quality cosmetics, hormonal depletion, immune suppression, and oxygen depletion can all contribute to leaving their marks upon our faces. Avoid squinting and frowning, as these will etch unnecessary lines in your face. Sugar consumption induces the collagen cross-linking that can cause wrinkles.

The skin of smokers ages up to twenty years faster than that of nonsmokers. The very act of smoking encourages wrinkles around the lips, crow's-feet, leathery skin quality, grayish color, and under-eye puffiness and discoloration. Also, the exposure to carbon monoxide reduces circulation by constricting blood vessels, resulting in drier, more wrinkled skin. Smoking impairs blood circulation to the skin and is a definite contributor to wrinkles, especially around the eye and lip areas. Every cigarette smoked destroys about 25 mg of vitamin C, which is needed for the production of collagen, our natural ally against wrinkles. And, of course, smoking causes us to squint when the smoke wafts in our faces. Yet after a person quits even long-term tobacco use, the skin's color and texture will improve.

Intense scrubbing and rubbing of the face can overstretch the skin, encouraging wrinkles. Repetitive facial movements and extreme facial expressions, such as frowning, squinting, wrinkling the nose, and propping your face in your hands, pull on the skin and weaken its supportive structure. Have a small hand mirror available and watch yourself speak on the phone sometime to observe just how many face-wrinkling movements you might be making. Purchase some cosmetic tape from a pharmacy, and when you have a few hours alone at home, apply the tape over your wrinkles. Or look for a product called Frownies (see Resources, page 229). Leave it on at night. (I try to do this after my husband has gone to bed and remove it before he wakes up. He gets to see me at my best.) This can alert you to the unnecessary facial movements you make so you can stop doing them. Use Frownies at least three times a week. Remove them gently by moistening them first. Splash your face with warm water, then moisturize.

People who smile are more likely to have smoother skin than those that frown constantly. When you smile, you only use thirteen muscles; frowning uses about sixty. Laughter also increases blood circulation to the skin and promotes a rosy glow.

Overconsumption of alcohol dilates the blood vessels, which can cause them to break; it also causes dehydration and depletes the body of nutrients, both of which contribute to wrinkles.

If the outer layer of skin becomes irritated or dry, the surface can become cracked and fine lines can appear. Overcleansing the face with harsh soaps that contain deodorants and detergents can strip the face of moisturizing oils. Soaps with oats and/or olive oil are the least drying. Better yet are gentle soap-free cleansers that are available with dry-skin-soothing ingredients, such as calendula. Apply a moisturizer right after cleansing, as water helps to keep the skin's outer layers from drying out and oil seals it in. During the day, rehydrate the skin with a mineral water spray, even over makeup. Drink at least eight to ten glasses of water. Reapply moisturizer faithfully. The keratinized protein of the top layers of skin requires water to look and feel supple.

Fruit, yogurt, and buttermilk contain the much touted alpha hydroxy acids that stimulate new cell growth; applied topically, they are humectant and promote younger-looking skin. You can make your own facial masks with mashed ripe fruits and vegetables such as avocado, banana, and carrot pulp. (See page 33 for information on how to make your own facial masks.) Essential oils that help fight wrinkles include chamomile, frankincense, lavender, and neroli; these essential oils can be found in many natural facial cleansers and moisturizers.

Remember to breathe more deeply and slowly. Avoid prolonged sun exposure. Humidify your home, especially during the winter months. Sleep on your back, as sleeping on your side or stomach causes facial creases that will lead to permanent lines. Sleep with an open window; not only does fresh air encourage sleep, it provides you with much-needed oxygen. Before bed, massage a small amount of serum into any lines you want to reduce; follow with a moisturizer. Acupressure and light massage can help move stagnated *chi*, which contributes to wrinkles. (See page 90 for directions on how to do facial acupressure.) Avoid resting your face in your hands, as this squishes your skin. Also avoid pressing your face into the telephone.

Eating high-quality unheated fats is essential. Moisture-rich foods include avocados, freshly ground flaxseeds, nuts, seeds, and winter squash. Also consume antioxidant-rich colorful fresh fruits and vegetables. Drink mineral-rich herbal teas made with marshmallow root, Irish moss, green tea, and violet leaves; be sure to also drink plenty of pure water. Vitamin C is necessary for collagen production. Vitamin E helps us utilize oxygen better, balances hormone production, and preserves the skin's elasticity. Zinc helps synthesize collagen and is essential for bringing dry, flaky skin back into balance. Gamma-linolenic acid (GLA) helps rebuild the skin's natural moisture barrier. Alpha lipoic acid inhibits glycation, or collagen cross-linking. Other supplements that may inhibit wrinkles include vitamin A, beta-carotene, pycnogenol, superoxide dismutase, and coenzyme Q10.

Antiwrinkle Exercises

- The Smile-Up exercise is a face-lifting technique. There are about fifty muscles in the face that control expression. These muscles usually occur in pairs. Draw an imaginary line, one-half inch away from the corners of your mouth to one-half inch away from the corners of your eyes. As these muscles are attached to most of the other muscles in the face, using these muscles can have a profound effect. Doing this exercise on a regular basis will make you look happier and have a toned appearance. Moisturize your face. Press the heels of your hands to the area on the outside of your eyes. Slightly elevate your chin and open your mouth about one inch. Lift your upper lip and cheek muscles at the same time, as if smiling hard, while also contracting your neck muscles. Hold for a count of seven. Repeat seven times.

- The zygomatic muscles stretch between the upper lip, over the cheekbones, and past the eyes. When they slacken, a line forms from the nose to the mouth (nasal labial fold). To diminish this line, place your thumb up and under the cheek area (via the mouth). Hold and massage in place, while you gently smile for a count of six. Repeat two times on each side.

- Crow's-feet are lateral creases at the outer edges of the eyes. Open your eyes wide and raise your eyebrows. With the heels of your hands keeping your brows raised, use your muscles to pull your brows down against your palms' resistance. Relax. Repeat six times.

Slant boards are a wonderful way to de-stress on a daily basis, and lying on one for ten to twenty minutes daily helps to prevent wrinkles by increasing circulation to the face; it also improves skin quality. I bought one as a present to myself a few years back and love it. However, anyone who has had a recent stroke should not use them, and those who have very high blood pressure or a detached retina should not try them without consulting with their physician first.

Now popular are acupuncture face-lifts. Long used by Chinese emperors to defy the appearance of aging, this safer, nonsurgical method to improving your appearance relaxes, supports, and strengthens muscles from inside.

Beauty tips can minimize the appearance of wrinkles while you work on improving your skin tone. Wear light-catching earrings to draw attention to the outer edges of your face. Light or white collars, silk scarves, and necklaces worn lower than the collarbone detract attention away from the face. Avoid dark lipsticks.

Mature skin can become more youthful with the use of the following herbs: calendula, comfrey leaf and root, marshmallow root, and rose. Essential oils that are of benefit include carrot seed, chamomile, cypress, fennel, frankincense, geranium, jasmine, lavender, myrrh, neroli, patchouli, rose, rose geranium, rosemary, and sandalwood.

Moisturizing Antiwrinkle Mister

Mist yourself several times daily for hydration and a feeling of freshness.

1/2 cup rose water

1/2 cup spring mineral water

Pour the ingredients into a clean plastic mister bottle. Shake before using. Spray on your face, with your eyes and mouth closed.

Dry Skin

As we age, our body will contain less water, more like 60 percent. Dry air can also contribute to even more dry skin. Skin that is excessively dry is more likely to wrinkle at an early age, though is less prone to enlarged pores and breakouts.

Seriously dry skin can be due to a depletion of fluids, and dry skin is especially prone to not being able to retain the moisture it has. The best way to hydrate the skin is from the inside; drinking at least a quart of pure water a day is essential. Though simply drinking water is not enough to cure dry skin, it does help the maintenance of interstitial fluids between the cells that contribute to forming a flexible matrix. Caffeine, alcohol, and tobacco are dehydrating to the skin. Skin care products such as soaps, cleansers, and alcohol-based products can contribute to drying out the skin. Weather, sun exposure, and the methods used to heat and cool our homes, cars, and workplaces can exacerbate dry-skin conditions. Estrogen helps the skin retain moisture by increasing the hyaluronic acid and mucopolysaccharide content in the skin; when menopause occurs, skin can retain less moisture. Lack of moisture causes a buildup of skin cells that adhere and prevent natural exfoliation and moisture retention. Skin can even get dried out from overuse of moisturizers that are so emollient that dead skin cells are held in place.

Good foods to eat more of to improve skin quality include the dark orange and green beta-carotene-rich foods like apricots, carrots, green leafy vegetables, parsley, pumpkin, sweet potatoes, and winter squash, as well as almonds, apples, avocados, barley, buckwheat, millet, oatmeal, pumpkin seeds, sesame seeds, sunflower seeds, and yogurt. It is also essential to consume the right kinds of fats. Get off commercial heated oils, such as soy, corn, and canola; these contain large amounts of omega-6 fatty acids, which contribute to inflammation. Instead, use skin-beautifying extra-virgin olive oil or raw coconut oil.

Dried-up skin lacks moistening *yin*, so drink moisturizing herbal teas, such as fennel seed, Irish moss, marshmallow root, plantain leaf, red clover blossoms, and violet leaves.

Since good skin health begins from within, various vitamins and minerals can be of benefit.

- **Vitamin A** helps to preserve the skin's elasticity, regulates sebaceous glands, protects against infection, and stimulates collagen formation. A deficiency may result in dry, itchy skin and make it more likely that dead skin cells will clog the pores, resulting in breakouts.
- **B-complex vitamins** help keep stress from showing its ravages on our skin. A deficiency is sometimes implicated in cracks around the mouth, corners of the mouth, and eyes.
- **Vitamin C** strengthens the capillaries, promotes healing, and increases skin elasticity.
- **Vitamin D** nourishes dry skin.
- **Vitamin E** helps the body utilize oxygen better, balances hormone production, and preserves elasticity.
- **Vitamin F** is often referred to as "the cosmetic vitamin." A deficiency can cause wrinkles, eczema, and thick dry skin.
- **Zinc** helps to synthesize collagen, boosts the immune system, and is essential for bringing dry, flaky skin into balance.

How we cleanse our skin can affect its moisture content. If you are using soap, avoid brands that contain deodorants and detergents. Soaps made of oatmeal, white clay, or olive oil are the least drying. Gentle cleansers are available with ingredients that are soothing to dry skin, such as vitamin E, oatmeal, coconut oil, and shea butter. Cleanse your face with warm (not hot) water, and rinse with at least ten splashes of cold water to remove any residue of cleanser. Certainly bathing and washing too often can dry out the skin.

Again, the best time to apply a moisturizer is right after cleansing, as water helps keep the skin's outer layers from drying out and oil seals it in. Avoid poor-quality cosmetics that contain mineral oil, chemicals, and artificial colors and fragrances.

Showers that are short and not too hot are less drying than baths. If you do like to soak in the tub, prepare a batch of rich bath oil made with two cups of cold-pressed coconut oil and one-half ounce of lavender essential oil. Shake the oils together and add two tablespoons to the bath.

You can also benefit your bathing with the addition of a mixture of moisturizing herbs tied into a washcloth and allowed to "steep" in the tub. Soothing herbs that feel and smell pleasant include the following:

- calendula
- chamomile flowers
- comfrey leaves
- elder blossoms
- fennel seed
- lavender flowers
- marshmallow root
- rosebuds
- violet leaves

However, herbs and oils can add a slippery quality to the bath, so be sure to have a bath mat and/or rail to avoid mishaps.

During the day, rehydrate your skin, especially your face, which is the part most exposed to the elements. A mister bottle may be filled with moistening ingredients and sprayed lightly with your eyes and mouth closed, even over makeup. You can fill the mister with a tea of chamomile, fennel, and/or orange blossoms. This should be kept refrigerated when not in use. One-half cup each of rose water and mineral water can be used as a moistening mist. Another easy spray can be made with eight ounces of water and ten drops of chamomile, geranium, lavender, neroli, and rose or sandalwood essential oil. Shake before spraying. If you fly in airplanes, keep in mind that cabin air is very drying and a spray mister is great to use for external hydration.

Natural Care for Dry Skin

THESE INGREDIENTS MAKE GOOD MASKS FOR DRY SKIN:

- apricot
- avocado
- banana
- oatmeal
- peach

HERBS TO MOISTEN DRY SKIN INCLUDE:

- calendula
- chamomile
- comfrey
- elder flowers
- linden flowers
- marshmallow

THESE ESSENTIAL OILS ALSO HELP DRY SKIN:

- bergamot
- cardamom
- carrot seed
- cedarwood
- chamomile
- champa
- clary sage
- fennel
- frankincense
- geranium
- jasmine
- juniper
- lavender
- lemon
- melissa
- myrrh
- neroli
- palmarosa
- patchouli
- peppermint
- rose
- rose geranium
- rosemary
- rosewood
- sage
- sandalwood
- vetivert
- ylang-ylang

Tips for Preventing Dry Skin

- Protect your skin from the elements, especially when outdoors between the hours of 10:00 a.m. and 4:00 p.m.
- Wear appropriate protective clothing.
- Stay clear of getting sunburned and avoid tanning booths.
- Exercise delivers oxygen and nutrients to the skin and increases collagen production.
- Avoid excessive heat, such as sitting close to the fire.
- Keep the heat lower in your house. Even here in Colorado, we turn it all the way off most nights in the winter. You'll not only save energy and reduce your power bill, you will also save your skin. Cold is a preservative.
- Smoking causes early wrinkles, yet even after long-term use and then quitting, the skin's color and texture will improve.
- Consider having a humidifier in the room, especially during the winter months when air becomes drier from heat sources.
- Plants in a room are especially moisturizing to the air and body.
- A good massage done with oil can be both relaxing and moisturizing.
- Wear natural-fiber clothing so your body can breathe! Polyester isn't too cool for many reasons. Fresh air is free medicine for the skin.
- Be aware that eczema, psoriasis, sun damage, rosacea, and early signs of skin cancer can resemble dry skin but are not benefited by regular moisturizers.

Face the world with a healthy-looking, moistened glow!

Oily Skin

Enlarged pores characterize oily skin, and excessive or excessively thick oil secretions exude from the sebaceous glands. Stress and hormones (due to pregnancy or birth control pills) can cause our skin to become suddenly oilier. Heredity, diet, cosmetics, humidity, and hot weather can all be factors. Oily skin is common in adolescence as hormone levels increase, particularly androgen, a male hormone that can be produced by the ovaries or adrenal glands, though oily skin can occur at any age. In general, skin tends to get drier with age.

The human body is the universe in miniature. That which cannot be found in the body is not to be found in the universe. Hence the philosopher's formula that the universe within reflects the universe without.

—MAHATMA GANDHI

Many people have skin that is oily in some areas but not others. This is considered combination skin. It is usually the T zone (forehead, nose and chin) that is most likely to be oily. The excess oil makes the skin more acid, shiny, thicker and more prone to blackheads and pimples. Pores are more likely to become clogged, making cleansing on a regular basis more necessary.

To determine if your skin is indeed oily, wash your face before bed but do not apply any moisturizers. In the morning, take five sheets of blotting paper (available in drugstores) and blot these areas separately: the chin, nose, cheeks, forehead, and hairline. Normal skin will show a small amount of oil. Dry skin will exhibit none. Oily skin will leave oil spots.

Seborrhea can occur wherever oil glands are plentiful: the scalp, sides of the nose, behind the ears, eyebrows and eyelids, midsection of the chest, arm folds, groin, breasts, and buttocks. Seborrhea can be due to excess oiliness, although it can also be caused by a type of fungal overgrowth.

One of the benefits of oily skin is that it is slower to show its age, though it can also be quicker to experience breakouts. To decrease the oiliness, include more apples, pears, plums, strawberries, watermelon, carrots, cucumbers, green leafy vegetables, and daikon radishes in your diet. Drinking plenty of water helps flush toxins from the body. Eat fewer fatty foods, such as fried foods, potato chips, ice cream, and dairy products, and reduce or eliminate foods made with refined grains, including breads and pasta. It sure makes sense to get off of heated oils and eat more fresh fruits and vegetables!

Beneficial herbal teas to consume to decrease skin oiliness include burdock root, chamomile flower, horsetail herb, oat straw, peppermint, thyme herb, white oak bark, witch hazel, and yarrow. A deficiency of vitamins B_2 and B_6 can contribute to excessive oiliness. Alpha lipoic acid can reduce pore size and inhibit bacterial growth.

Avoid super-rich soaps that contain coconut oil, milky and creamy cleansers, or cleansers that don't use water. Too much skin washing can increase oil production. Hot water helps break up oil better than lukewarm water. Use a mild, nonabrasive exfoliant twice a week to keep pores from getting clogged. Be careful of overusing scrubs that can stimulate overactive oil glands. A clay mask twice a week can also be helpful.

Witch hazel or plain aloe vera juice can be applied after cleansing. Try using a toner that is alcohol free. Applying a light, oil-free moisturizer can encourage the skin to produce less oil. Keep your hands and hair off of your face to avoid transferring dirt, oil, and bacteria. If you use makeup, use only water-based products rather than ones that contain oil.

Natural Care for Oily Skin

ESSENTIAL OILS TO USE IN FACIAL SPRAYS:

- basil
- bergamot
- camphor
- cedarwood
- clove
- cypress
- eucalyptus
- frankincense
- geranium
- juniper
- lavender
- lemon
- melissa
- neroli
- orange
- sage
- sandalwood
- tea tree
- vetivert

HERBS FOR FACIAL STEAMS:

- elder flower
- horsetail herb
- lemongrass
- licorice root
- peppermint leaf
- rose flowers
- sage leaf
- witch hazel bark
- yarrow herb

Essential oils can help regulate the sebaceous glands, but they need to be diluted. One lovely method is to create a facial spray. Herbs can be used topically as facial steams and in commercial products for oily skin. Essential oils and herbs for oily skin are listed in the box on the previous page.

A couple of homeopathic remedies to decrease oily skin include:

- ***Mercurius*** improves oily skin that is accompanied by an unpleasant odor. The oiliness tends to be worse during cold and hot weather.
- ***Natrum muriaticum*** helps oily, shiny skin that is worse on hairy areas of the body. The person tends to be constipated.

Enlarged Pores

A pore is an opening on the surface of the skin that allows oil to escape. When the lungs and spleen are weak, pores are more likely to be enlarged.

There are several folk remedies that can give temporary relief to enlarged pores. Grind almonds into a powder to use as a gentle scrub. A facial mask of honey or puréed fresh tomato can be left on for twenty minutes then rinsed off. Apply cucumber juice, witch hazel, or buttermilk as a toner after cleansing. Taking vitamin C daily improves the function of oil-secreting glands.

Pore-Minimizing Toner

Use this to minimize the appearance of pores.

1/4 cup rose water

1 teaspoon witch hazel

Combine the ingredients in a clean bottle. Use to mist your face (with eyes and mouth closed), or apply with a cotton ball.

Acne

It is indeed difficult when acne causes us to make a poor first impression and our health issues are so publicly announced on our face. Acne, also known as acne vulgaris or simply pimple outbreaks, is an inflammation of the skin that results from clogged pores. Acne is likely to occur when sebum, a waxy substance that lubricates the skin, and keratin, a skin protein, block the sebaceous glands. Acne is the body's immune response, sending lymph to an inflamed area, which also causes swelling and a pimple.

Acne can have many causes: Allergies, poor circulation, constipation, food sensitivities, medications, nutritional deficiencies, smoking, stress, yeast overgrowth, inadequate sloughing off of the skin's cells, overactive oil glands, and lack of fatty acids (which reduce inflammation). Excess sebum production can be partly genetic or hormonal; acne is most likely to occur on oily skin. Stress can cause the skin to produce more oil. However, dry, flaky skin can clog pores and contribute to acne. If there is excess or irregular dead-skin-cell shedding, pores can get clogged, which may lead to breakouts.

A buildup of bacteria (especially *Propionibacterium acnes*) in the pores can also cause breakouts. As *P. acnes* reproduces, inflammation and irritation occur, causing many breakouts to be red and swollen. The bacteria that contribute to acne are anaerobic, which means they do not thrive well in the presence of oxygen. That's another reason to breathe deeply, get plenty of fresh air and exercise, and eat lots of green leafy oxygen-transporting vegetables!

Hormonal fluctuations, especially excessive levels of the hormone androgen (which is at its highest level right before menstruation begins), may be a contributing factor. Androgen and testosterone, both male sex hormones (found also in women, but to a much lesser degree), becomes active around puberty and stimulate larger quantities of sebum, which can contribute to clogged pores and result in pimples and acne. In adults over age twenty-five, food allergies are often a culprit in skin breakouts. Acne can sometimes begin with the onset of menopause.

Acne is considered a "damp heat condition" in Asian medicine. To remedy acne, improve lymphatic flow and blood circulation, and reduce the amount of sebum produced, it is important to keep all the channels of elimination open, such as the colon, lungs, kidneys, and liver, so they can do their job of purifying the body so pimples don't end up on your skin. The liver helps break down an overabundance of hormones; a poorly functioning liver can make the skin go haywire.

Blemishes are simply common skin imperfections. In Asian medicine, "Liver acne" is said to be singular, large, ugly pimples, while "Kidney acne" consists of crops of reddish pimples; pustules (inflamed red, raised bumps that contain pus) are possible with either of these. Cystic acne consists of blackheads, whiteheads, papules (inflamed red, raised bumps that do not contain pus), pustules, and nodules (hardened bumps). This type of acne is the most likely to scar. When hair follicles become encrusted with dead skin buildup, hard tiny bumps can occur, especially on the thighs and upper arms; this is known as *keratosis pilaris*.

Blackheads

The mildest form of acne manifests as blackheads and whiteheads, also known as milia, which are hard white bumps that are not red or swollen and do not contain pus. If an inflamed pore's surface is covered by skin, it is a whitehead.

If the pore is open and doesn't have skin covering it, and the top is exposed to air, it darkens and becomes a blackhead.

A blackhead is composed of sebum, bacteria, and dead cells. The dark color of a blackhead is oxidized sebum, not dirt. By the time a blackhead is visible, it could have been months in development.

Do facial steams twice a week. Good herbs to include in the steam include elder flowers and rosemary. Gently massaging baking soda into the skin helps sebum escape. A gentle scrub of almond meal or cornmeal with a complexion brush can also be used. Honey, oatmeal, and tomato masks improve blackheads.

When left alone, blackheads and whiteheads usually clear up on their own. Squeezing them can bruise and deepen the damage. If you are going to attempt to squeeze out a blackhead (even though you know you shouldn't), the best time is after doing a facial steam or after having applied a hot wet compress to the area first. This is to ensure that the pores are soft and open. With a clean piece of cotton or tissue, squeeze upward and outward. If it doesn't want to come out easily, stop; otherwise, irritation can occur, leaving you with a bigger problem. Afterward, apply some lavender or tea tree essential oil or distilled witch hazel.

By the time an imperfection shows up on the skin, it may have been in the making for two or three weeks. Acne begins in the pores or hair follicles. Though it frequently occurs on the face, the chest, shoulders, and back are also susceptible due to their high concentration of oil glands.

It is always good to consider any emotional implications in acne, such as not accepting oneself, anger, frustration, holding on to past hurts, and feeling picked on during childhood. When we are in a messy life situation, our skin tries to "break out" of that situation. Stress, depression, and anxiety can worsen acne. Process these feelings in a safe, positive, and effective way—try journaling, talking to a trusted friend, or enlisting the help of a therapist.

Consider changing your pillowcase every other night. Wash your hands frequently during the day, and avoid touching your face unnecessarily (and when you must touch your face, use only clean hands). Keep your hair off your face and be aware that hair products, such as sprays, gels, and mousses, can contain pore-clogging ingredients. Keep in mind that holding a telephone receiver against your face can put your skin in contact with bacteria that cause acne. Wipe down your phone with alcohol daily.

Picking, squeezing, and digging at pimples may be difficult to resist but can create more damage, scabs, and scars. Squeezing pimples breaks fine capillaries and causes skin damage. When you feel a pimple erupting, rather than squeezing it, apply spirits of camphor or lavender, cedarwood, neem, or tea tree essential oil four or five times daily to dry it up. Tea tree oil has a similar effect to benzoyl peroxide. Apply it only to the area where you want to dry up a pimple.

If you feel you must squeeze, do so only after a pimple has formed a head. First cleanse the skin, then place a cloth soaked in hot water over the area.

Cover each finger with a tissue to prevent slippage, and apply soft, even pressure on the sides of the pimple, gently pressing down, then up around the area. Do this only once or twice. If nothing gets released, continuing to press will only traumatize and damage more skin. Afterward, apply a spot of lavender or tea tree oil to the area. If you are prone to scarring, use an ointment containing vitamin E, calendula, and comfrey once the pimple is in the drying stage.

Cleanse your skin with a water-soluble cleanser that will not clog your pores. Antibacterial soaps can be too harsh and drying. Thick products, such as creams, are more likely to be pore congesting. Facial steams can be done twice weekly. Avoid excessive exfoliation and harsh granular scrubs, which can stimulate oil glands that are already overactive. Facial masks to use when dealing with acne can be made of honey, powdered rolled oats, ripe pineapple, grated raw potato, or tomato. Apply witch hazel or aloe vera as a toner after cleansing.

Foods for Acne

Acne is best treated with diet and exercise. The foods that are most beneficial for improving acne include raw almonds, apples, apricots, artichokes, barley, beets, carrots (with the skins), celery, cucumbers (organic, with the peel), flaxseeds, green leafy vegetables, lemon in water, parsley, radishes, sweet potatoes, raw sunflower seeds, and winter squashes. A high-fiber raw diet, free of heated oils, refined carbohydrates, dairy, sugar, and wheat, is the ultimate.

Foods to minimize include oranges and grapefruits, hot spicy foods, peanuts, peanut butter, wheat, excess nuts (except for almonds), high-fat dairy products, sugar, hydrogenated fats, heated oils (including commercially bottled salad dressing and oils like canola, soy, and safflower oil), and fried foods. Oil that is heated for frying and other types of cooking goes into the air and can clog the pores. The hormones that are added to commercial dairy products and meats can overstress the liver, as it will be forced to not only metabolize our own hormones but those fed to the animals as well. Dairy products can contain high levels of progesterone, and commercial meats can carry a wide variety of hormones, including steroids and thyroid-releasing hormones. Some people with acne are sensitive to the iodine in shellfish. Of course, not everyone has sensitivities to the same foods or product ingredients.

Herbs and Remedies for Acne Care

Teas or tinctures that help reduce skin eruptions are made from combinations of burdock root, raw dandelion root, milk thistle seed, Oregon grape root, red clover blossom, sarsaparilla root, and yellow dock root. Drink plenty of fluids and herbal tea. For hormonally related acne, use chaste tree berry internally. A daily capsule of turmeric powder can help clear up skin breakouts. Natural food stores carry capsules and tinctures that include combinations of several of these herbs. Select your product and use it three times daily. You could also make up a tea blend with these herbs.

Herbs that benefit acne-prone skin, and which are found in many natural body care products, include calendula, comfrey, and elder flowers. Acne-prone skin may be helped by body care products that contain one or more of the essential oils listed in the box at the right.

The homeopathic remedy *Sulphur 30c* taken three times daily can sometimes help clear up acne.

Essential Oils for Acne-Prone Skin

- bergamot
- cajeput
- camphor
- cedarwood
- chamomile
- cypress
- eucalyptus
- fir
- geranium
- grapefruit
- juniper
- lavender
- lemon
- lemongrass
- myrrh
- neroli
- naiouli
- palmarosa
- rosemary
- rosewood
- sandalwood
- tea tree
- yarrow
- ylang-ylang

Nutrients and Enzymes for Acne Care

- Vitamin A helps reduce sebum and is a natural antioxidant.
- B-complex vitamins can help regulate hormones, especially B_6, which can help calm the raging hormones of teenaged girls during menstrual flare-ups.
- Niacin, also known as vitamin B_3, is a vasodilator. Although it may make you feel hot, red, itchy, and prickly for about ten minutes, it does so much to increase the amount of nutrients and oxygen transported to the skin. It also removes wastes, which can help clear up difficult skin conditions such as acne. Try taking 100 mg of niacin daily. Niacin should be avoided by those with rosacea, couperose conditions, and very thin, sensitive skin.
- Vitamin C improves white blood cell function, helps the body resist infection, and is an antioxidant.
- Vitamin E is an antioxidant that helps the body better utilize the retinol in vitamin A.
- Essential fatty acids help dissolve fatty deposits that congest the pores.
- Chromium helps regulate blood sugar levels.
- Selenium helps increase glutathione peroxidase, an enzyme that is usually at very low levels in those with acne.
- If zinc is deficient, then sebaceous glands can become enlarged.
- MSM is a form of sulfur that inhibits bacterial growth and promotes more rapid healing.
- A probiotic supplement (such as acidophilus) helps detoxify the gastrointestinal tract and decrease unfriendly organisms like *Candida*.

- Digestive enzymes can make the skin more resistant to bacteria and improve the digestive disorders that can contribute to acne. Lipase is an enzyme that helps the body better metabolize fats and can be very helpful.

For more ideas on managing acne, see the sections on cleansing (page 29), facial steams (page 32), masks (page 33), and toners (page 44).

Scars

Skin has an amazing ability to heal and regenerate. In general, there are three stages of skin healing. In the first stage, a scab forms and is often accompanied by tenderness, swelling, and redness. During the next stage, new skin is forming underneath the scab as the body produces collagen and re-forms what constitutes the intercellular matrix. The last stage is where the inner and outer layers of skin rebuild. As time passes, the scab decreases, redness and inflammation are reduced, and the skin hopefully returns to normal. New scars are easier to minimize than older scars. Indented scars are below the skin. Keloid scars are lumpy, protruding, and raised.

Many scars could be prevented if we all knew how to take care of wounds, though some scarring tendencies are genetic. Allow the skin to breathe as much as possible. If a bandage must be used, make sure it is breathable, or use gauze with tape only at the sides of the wound. Remove any coverings at night, if possible. Keep the damaged area clean, but don't overclean. A small amount of aloe vera gel can be applied for its biogenic-stimulating properties. Heavy creams used early on will prevent the wounded area from getting adequate oxygen. After the wound has healed somewhat, applying products to promote healing, such as aloe vera, avocado oil, calendula flowers, castor oil, cocoa butter, comfrey, honey, plantain, and shea butter, will help to treat and prevent scars. Keep using these after the scab has gone. Avoid heavy, pore-clogging creams, synthetic fragrances, and harsh cleansers. Scars are best treated when they are newer, but calendula, castor oil, and plantain have helped even old scars. Scars can take from several months to two years to heal. Alpha hydroxy acid (AHA) peels or laser resurfacing can help reduce any scar that is persistent. Avoid getting lots of sun with a wound that has the potential for scarring, as it can render the scar more permanent. Picking at scabs can cause scarring that might not have occurred otherwise.

If there is the potential for a scar, consume foods rich in beta-carotene and vitamins E and B complex. Especially good are apples, apricots, cucumbers, millet, rice, rye, apricots, and sea vegetables. Vegetable juices made with diluted carrot, celery, endive, lemon, and pineapple juice can be consumed.

Vitamin E, used both internally and topically, is a favorite remedy for preventing scars. Taking alpha lipoic acid, zinc, vitamin C, and bromelain internally may also help prevent and treat scar formation.

Use a salve containing vitamin E, aloe vera, calendula, plantain, and castor oil. Good essential oils that help heal and prevent scars include frankincense, geranium, lavender, and neroli.

Homeopathic Remedies for Scars

- ***Causticum*** is best for deep scars and old injuries that still feel sore.
- ***Crocus*** helps heal old wounds that still open.
- ***Fluoric acid*** benefits old scars that become red around the edges. It can also help keloid scars.
- ***Graphites*** can help minimize old, hard scars.
- ***Kali iodatum*** is the remedy for scars that are the remains of small boils on the face, scalp, neck, chest, and back.
- ***Lachesis*** is a classic remedy for scars that bleed and break open easily.
- ***Phytolacca*** is used when all else fails.
- ***Silicea*** helps scars that remain from boils or ulcers, as well as keloid scars.

Stretch Marks

Stretch marks are a common aftermath of pregnancy. Lubricate your body daily to help prevent stretch marks. Be sure to oil the perineal area, belly, hips, thighs, and breasts, which are all areas where stretch marks can occur. This is especially important the last three months of pregnancy so your skin will be supple and will stretch during delivery. Even plain coconut oil can be used.

Pregnant Belly Butter

Love your baby and your body with this blend.

2 cups olive or coconut oil
1/2 ounce calendula flowers, crushed
1/2 ounce comfrey leaves, crushed
1 tablespoon vitamin E oil
5 drops lavender essential oil

Place the crushed herbs and olive oil in a dry, clean glass jar. Allow to steep for two weeks. Strain through a clean, dry cotton cloth while squeezing the oil out of the herbs. Discard the herbs. Stir in the vitamin E and lavender oil. Bottle. Apply to areas prone to stretching at least twice daily.

Discolorations

Liver spots are also known as age spots, sun spots, lentigines, solar lentigos, and senile keratosis. They are changes in the skin's pigmentation, usually of light to dark brown coloring, or light to dark gray, that may appear on the face, neck, V of the neck, and backs of the hands. Though they often come on as we age, aging does not have to be the cause.

Age spots can be brought on through nutritional deficiencies, free radical damage, elevated blood sugar levels, sun exposure, and topical alcohol contact (such as cologne and some cosmetics). Another causative factor can be cross-linking of the skin cells (which can be caused by sun exposure, cigarette smoke, fatty foods, alcohol, and/or smog). Asian medicine does ascribe liver imbalances as the cause.

Drink lemon and water daily. Eat fresh raw leafy greens daily. Get off of heated oils. Use foods high in beta-carotene; B complex (especially folic acid and niacin); vitamins C and E; zinc; superoxide dismutase; glutathione; cystine; and pycnogenol.

Lemon juice, fresh pineapple, chamomile tea, dandelion leaf, yogurt, castor oil, shea butter, buttermilk, and elder flower water all have lightening effects when applied regularly to the skin. Daily exfoliations with powdered rolled oats and yogurt can also help remove discolorations. Vitamin E oil mixed with lemon essential oil can also help.

Protect the skin from the sun, even if it means wearing a hat and cotton gloves. I do know that I had many of these spots before going raw, and now I barely have any!

Skin Lightening Formula

Try this for freckles and age spots. After a few weeks, you should see some lightening.

- 1/4 cup chopped fresh dandelion leaves
- 4 tablespoons castor oil

Steep the leaves in the oil for 2 weeks. Strain. Use daily.

Skin Lightening Treatment

This one is my favorite for lightening age spots or melasma.

- 1/2 cup ripe papaya
- 1 tablespoon freshly squeezed lemon juice
- 1 teaspoon raw honey

Mash all the ingredients in a bowl. Apply to the areas you want to lighten. Leave on for 5 minutes, then rinse.

Freckles

Though freckles do have their charm, skin that is likely to freckle is associated with deficiencies in vitamins A and E. Topical applications of aloe vera, buttermilk, yogurt, lemon juice (mixed with 50 percent water), mashed grapes, parsley, or elder flower water have been traditionally used. Do minimize sun exposure.

A Folk Remedy for Freckles

1 cup water

1/2 cup rose water

1/4 cup yogurt

1 teaspoon boric acid

Combine all the ingredients in a blender and process until smooth. Dab on the freckles before bedtime. Stored in the refrigerator, it will keep for about a month.

Cellulite

Cellulite is sometimes called "orange peel skin" or "hail damage." The French word for cellulite literally translates to "cell inflammation." Cellulite is actually a combination of fat, water, and metabolic wastes. It is not a serious health threat, but its existence can prevent nourishment from reaching the cells. It is one of the many forms of blocked *chi*.

As we age, our connective fibers become thinner, and underlying pockets of fat bulge through the cell walls. The rippling effect is due to fluid retention in the adipose (fatty) tissue. These trapped fluids contain toxins and cause swelling, creating a blockage that decreases the ability of nutrients, oxygen, and blood to circulate through the body. This contributes to the breakdown of collagen and elastin fibers. Poor elimination, lymph congestion, increase in fatty tissue, fluid retention, poor posture, sedentary jobs, shallow breathing, heredity, and lack of exercise are all contributing factors to this stagnant condition.

Cellulite usually resides along the buttocks, hips, and thighs, in the subcutaneous tissue along with the fat cells. These areas have few connective fibers but lots of underlying fat. Together, they form a "honeycomb" of dimpled skin that keeps fat in place.

Even men and thin women can have cellulite. Varicose veins are also more likely when cellulite impairs circulation. Good cellular metabolism, an active circulatory system, better lymphatic movement, and better elimination of toxins are all necessary to eliminate cellulite. Unfortunately, it won't automatically disappear with diet and exercise.

Breathe more deeply and fully. Practice good posture. As you walk, stretch the areas affected by cellulite. Do leg and hip exercises regularly. Callanetics exercises can be helpful as they work very deeply. Do leg exercises in the pool or tub to tighten hips and thighs. Other beneficial exercises include running, bicycling, skating, dancing, and swimming.

Remember the "bicycle exercise"? While lying on your back, elevate your legs and hips perpendicular to your torso. Place a pillow under your lower back, and pedal as if you were riding a bicycle. Try this for ten minutes daily. "Hot yoga!" says my best friend, Tamara.

Let go of any old hurts. Clean out clutter in your home. Let go of what no longer serves.

Improve digestion so your body can better metabolize water and fat. Eat more fresh fruits and vegetables, especially apples, asparagus, string beans, cabbage, carrots, fennel, grapefruit, lettuce, papayas, pineapples, radishes, spinach, strawberries, tomatoes, turnips, and watercress. A diet rich in natural vitamin C will promote collagen health.

Avoid fried foods, red meat, foods with animal hormones, heated fats, sugar, salt, and refined carbohydrates. Drink lots more water. Lemon in water is always good. Drink a tablespoon of unpasteurized apple cider vinegar in water each morning.

Try dry brush skin massage (see page 40) using extra pressure in the areas where cellulite exists. In the bath or shower, do salt scrubs (see page 42). Use circular kneading (like dough) strokes, deeply massaging with your knuckles up and down vertically, and chopping, percussion-like strokes. You can even massage fresh mashed kiwi or pineapple into your skin. Alternatively, use coconut oil scented with any of the following essential oils: bergamot, black pepper, cypress, eucalyptus, fennel, geranium, ginger, grapefruit, juniper, lemon, orange, oregano, peppermint, rosemary, sage, tangerine, or vetivert. Enjoy professional massages.

Adding sea vegetables to your baths and using body wraps are good hydrotherapy techniques. Using a showerhead, alternate between hot and cold water for thirty seconds each, always beginning with hot and ending with cold. Use a loofah, ayate cloth, bristle brush, or mitt in the shower.

Herbs to use internally include butcher's broom, gotu kola, hawthorn, and horse chestnut cream. Sea vegetables can be used as a food, condiment, and herb.

Anti-Cellulite Massage Oil

Massage this blend into areas where you want to break up stuck energy.

- 1/8 cup cold-pressed coconut oil, at room temperature
- 3 drops cypress essential oil
- 3 drops geranium essential oil
- 3 drops grapefruit essential oil
- 3 drops juniper essential oil
- 3 drops rosemary essential oil

Place all the ingredients in a jar and shake well before applying to the skin.

Varicose Veins

Veins carry carbon dioxide–filled blood back to the heart and lungs and must defy gravity in order to make that trip. Veins are rather fragile, and any defective vein wall can result in dilation and damage to the valves, which can cause pressure and bulging veins. It is the veins on the sides of the legs, upper parts of the calves, and inner thighs just under the skin that are most likely to be affected by varicosities. Men can get varicose veins as well as women, though women are about four times more likely to be affected.

Normally, blood flows into the veins after it has deposited its nutrients into the capillaries and returns to the heart so it can be reoxygenated. There are one-way valves in the legs that help move the blood upward against the pull of gravity. The longest distance blood has to travel is from the feet to the heart. Most of the blood will be shunted upward, though if a lot remains and pools in the legs it can cause dilation and damage.

Symptoms of varicose veins include cramping; dull, aching pain; heavy feeling in the legs; swollen ankles; and itching, tingling, and burning sensations in the skin of the legs. Symptoms may manifest before the varicosities are apparent. Spider veins, also known as telangiectasias, are overgrown dilated blood vessels and are usually found on the calves and upper thighs.

Varicosities can result from sun damage, puberty, pregnancy, birth control pills, hormone replacement drugs, prolonged heat exposure (such as to hot tubs and saunas or standing in front of a hot oven), pressure, smoking, and injury. Obesity and old age put us at greater risk. Lack of muscle mass and tissue tone can cause veins to weaken. Varicose veins may be worse for women around their menstrual cycle, especially for those who retain fluids. Heredity can make us more likely candidates, and those with such tendencies must do their best to prevent them before they occur. If the liver and kidneys are unhealthy and unable to clean the blood, they can also contribute to varicose veins. If the connective tissue that supports the veins is weak, this also poses a risk.

Feeling overworked or overburdened or not being able to stand up for oneself can be contributing psychological factors. If you have a secret desire to kick someone, kick a pillow to relieve tension.

When a person stands for long periods of time or does lots of heavy lifting, pressure in the veins increases. Therefore, people with occupations that require standing in one place are put at a higher risk for varicose veins. It is better to be active and walk or bike ride, which moves pooled blood back into the circulatory system.

To help prevent varicosities, avoid long periods of sitting, especially with your legs crossed or folded beneath you. If you must cross your legs (because your mom told you to), do so at the ankles, not the knees. Elevate your legs when sitting, if possible. If you have a desk job, adjust your chair so that there is not a lot of pressure on the backs of your thighs. Sit on the floor with your legs stretched in front of you whenever possible (for instance, when watching a movie on television). If you must sit or stand for long periods of time, wiggle your toes and flex and rotate your feet. Rise up on your toes and slowly sink to your heels. You can also practice isometric exercises by tightening your muscles and then relaxing them. Do deep knee bends and a short walk when taking a break instead of drinking another cup of coffee.

Wearing tight clothes, such as tight pants, girdles, or socks with tight elastic bands, will impair circulation. Wearing support hose, however, can help relieve the discomfort of varicosities.

Elevate your bed four to six inches by putting blocks under the foot of your bed, or put a pillow under your ankles to elevate your legs slightly. Instead of jumping out of bed in the morning and applying sudden pressure on your legs, stay in bed a few minutes and stretch and flex your legs and feet before slowly getting up.

Regular exercise helps to strengthen muscle tone and improve circulation. Brisk walking, Rollerblading, aerobic dancing, swimming, cross-country skiing, and biking are all excellent activities for those who are prone to varicose veins. Do your best to avoid walking on paved surfaces, and choose more natural, uneven places to promenade so that you use a wider variety of muscles. The old high school gym exercise "bicycling," where you lay on your back, elevate your hips and legs, and make a pedaling motion is also excellent. Slant boards elevate the feet above the heart (see the Resources section on page 229). Those who are adept can practice the yoga shoulderstand daily.

Varicosities are rare in parts of the world where a high-fiber diet is consumed. When fiber is lacking, people are more likely to be constipated and tend to strain during bowel elimination, which puts pressure on the veins. Eat more vegetables (especially dark leafy greens, beets, cabbage, okra, and sea vegetables) and salads. Use raw purslane, which is a rich source of omega-3 fatty acids. Add plenty of garlic, onions, and small amounts of cayenne to your food to improve circulation. Whole grains that are beneficial to the circulatory system include barley, buckwheat, and oats. Eat fruits high in bioflavonoids, such as blueberries and cherries.

Juices to include are beet, carrot, celery, cucumber, parsley, spinach, and wheatgrass. Avoid consuming heated oils so you don't create viscous blood. Red meat, dairy products, fried foods, margarine, and hydrogenated oils do not pave the path to beauty. Be sure to drink plenty of fluids.

A supplement of vitamin C with bioflavonoids, quercetin, and rutin helps to strengthen the capillaries. Vitamin E helps the blood utilize oxygen better and prevents blood clots. MSM improves healing time and reduces inflammation.

Herbs to treat varicose veins include the following:

- **Bilberry** and **butcher's broom** strengthen weak capillaries.
- **Bu zhong yi qi wan** is a patented Chinese formula (sold as Central Qi Pills) for varicosities that tonify the spleen (which helps the blood stay in the proper channels) and improve liver function.
- **Ginkgo** helps to relax blood vessels and improve peripheral circulation.
- **Horse chestnut** is used both internally and topically to reduce swelling and strengthen the veins.
- **Nettle** improves circulation, nourishes the blood, and improves the elimination of toxins.

Some homeopathic remedies to relieve varicose veins include:

- ***Arsenicum album*** is for swelling, burning sensations, and possible ulcerations. Use for varicosities that feel relief from heat.
- ***Calcarea carbonica*** is for varicosities without pain. Use for overweight people with cold feet who feel worse from overexertion.
- ***Fluoric acid*** helps varicose ulcers and burning pain, especially where the left leg is most affected.
- ***Hamamelis virginica*** is a classic remedy where the legs are swollen and tender to touch. The person feels worse from walking or standing, and during pregnancy, yet better from cold.
- ***Pulsatilla*** helps inflammation and stinging pain. It is also used for those who feel worse during pregnancy.
- ***Sepia*** helps relieve varicosities that have occurred since pregnancy.

If the varicosities cause pain or discomfort, a moist warm compress of mullein, sage, white oak bark, and witch hazel or yarrow tea can be applied loosely to the area. A cabbage leaf or apple cider vinegar compress can also be applied and left on overnight.

Avoid deep massage atop a varicose vein, as loosening a blood clot may be dangerous. However, gently applying some arnica oil to the area can gradually help disperse congestion. Do this only on unbroken skin. At night, alternate hot and cold foot baths, beginning with hot water and ending with cold.

When the veins are near the surface, they are more of a cosmetic problem than a health threat. However, blockage of deeper veins can lead to thrombophlebitis, pulmonary embolism, stroke, or myocardial infarction.

If a rash or ulceration appears on the skin, it may indicate a condition more serious than surface varicosities and should be checked by a competent health professional. If ulcerations occur, a salve or poultice of chickweed, comfrey, or liquid chlorophyll may be applied.

Varicose Vein Soothing Oil

Massage this very gently into areas that are troubled by varicosities, as deep massage in these areas can loosen a blood clot.

- 1/2 cup coconut oil
- 40 drops rosemary essential oil
- 40 drops juniper essential oil
- 20 drops lemon essential oil

Combine all the ingredients and use to massage over the legs.

THE BEAUTIFUL PLEASURES OF THE BATH

There's no place like a bath to stretch your soul and listen to your own inner voice.

—SENECA

Hydrotherapy is the term for therapeutic treatments using water; it was practiced by the Babylonians, Egyptians, Greeks, and Romans. Drinking and bathing are also part of hydrotherapy. The word "spa," often scrawled as graffiti on ancient public baths, is from the Latin *saludis per aqua*, which means "health through water." Go visit local hot springs. Gathering at hot springs with families, friends, and lovers is a wonderful idea to help heal on many levels. And, of course, healthy relations radiate beauty. Ending a hot bath with a cold shower is great hydrotherapy to improve skin tone, feel invigorated, and stimulate the immune system. It is one of the best ways to get stronger.

Water is by far our most valuable cosmetic. Soaking in a warm, fragrant tub can be a sensual delight, offering time to retreat, reflect, and refresh. A bath taken right when you come home from work can make you more pleasant to be around. However, if you take a bath in the middle of the day and expect to get any work done, make it cooler and shorter, or you might be too relaxed to accomplish much else with your day. It is best to bathe at least a couple of hours after a big meal, to avoid interfering with digestion. Baths before bed aid sleep, as they elevate the body's temperature and the body will compensate by lowering its temperature, thus making us ready for sleep.

Showers that are short and not too hot are considered less drying than baths. In the United States, the average shower uses 25 to 75 gallons of water. In a shower, we have to stand up, so the experience is less relaxing. However, if you are particularly dirty, sweaty, or sticky, consider taking a short cleansing shower before submerging into a relaxing bath. For people who can't stand up, a beach chair can be placed in a tub to make showering or a sponge bath easier. Consider installing a shower filter or a whole-house water filter to limit chemical exposure.

Keep your bathroom clean so it can be a place to relax, refresh, and purify. A bath mat on the inside and outside of the tub can help you to keep from slipping and getting injured. Bath pillows, loofahs, fluffy towels, scented soaps, and candlelight all add to the serenity of the bathing experience. Relaxing music calms the soul, but avoid any electrical dangers. A bowl of washed grapes or some organic juice in a nonbreakable goblet can bring added delight.

Bath temperatures that are too hot are drying and can make you feel weak. Keep the temperature between 75 and 98 degrees, depending on the season. If you are taking a hot bath as therapy, you can wear a turban soaked in cool water. Very hot baths should be avoided during pregnancy or in cases of stomach ulcers, high blood pressure, or inflammation, or during excessive menstrual flow. If you ever feel faint during a bath, rather than stand, splash your face and body with cool water. A final cold rinse will energize you. A cold bath can be used to energize, lower a high fever, reduce pain, calm spasms, or treat constipation. A bath should not last much more than twenty minutes or your skin will start to wrinkle. A bath is an excellent place to enjoy a facial mask or a deep-conditioning treatment for your hair.

We don't want to waste resources, so it's not necessary to fill the tub too high. Placing a warm wet washcloth on your chest area can help infuse warmth throughout your body. If you use natural products, you could even collect some of the "gray water" to water the garden.

Most bubble baths contain sodium laurel sulfate, which dissolves the natural oils of the skin. Bubble baths and foaming bath gels can also leave a coating on the skin that must be rinsed off. Bath beads are often made of chemical salt compounds, mineral oil, and synthetic fragrances. Avoid using commercial potpourris in the bath. Many have synthetic fragrances that may irritate the skin. Soap can interfere with the healing properties of herbs or aromatherapy oils used in the bath. Taking a shower first to get clean before an aromatherapy bath is an excellent way to maximize the benefits of essential oils.

To use herbs or other dry substances, such as rolled oats, for the bath, simply tie a handful of the fresh or dried herbs or grain into a washcloth and secure it closed with a hair tie. Use a dark cloth so you don't stain your light-colored ones. If you have a stash of clean lost "single" socks, those also work great for bath bags. Use the herb-filled cloth to scrub your body as you deeply inhale the benefits. To keep your plumbing from getting clogged, don't allow bulky material to go down the drain. If you have used items that are floating loose and are not enclosed, such as sea vegetables or fresh flowers, be sure to use the metal filter when draining the tub. The spent flower and plant material can then be composted.

Alternatively, you could make a strong herbal tea with about one-half cup of herbs. Simmer it gently for twenty minutes, and then strain the tea into the tub. Another option is to throw a few ready-made tea bags into the bath. Liquids, such as apple cider vinegar (about 1 cup), or salts (1 pound) that dissolve readily can simply be added to the bath.

An even easier way to prepare the bath would be to use five to ten drops of pure essential oil as a substitute for the desired herb (although not all herbs are available as essential oils). Essential oils can also be mixed into a carrier oil to disperse, then added to the bath. (If too much essential oil is added, it could burn the skin. If this happens, wash off the essential oil and apply vegetable oil directly to the skin.) For example, you could make a bath with lavender flowers, either in a sock or a tea, or you could simply add lavender essential oil to the bath. Add essential oils after filling the tub so the fragrance does not dissipate before you get in. Close the curtain to hold in steam. Turn off the water while you floss, brush, or check e-mail. When the bath has cooled to a comfortable temperature, get into it. If you choose to use any citrus products, such as lemon peel or orange essential oil, use them at night, as they can make your skin more photosensitive. If you want to use fresh or dried citrus peels, be sure they are organic if they will be in contact with your skin.

For a hot tub, add three drops of essential oil per person. Consider eucalyptus, lavender, or tea tree oil.

Therapeutic Baths

- **Apple Cider Vinegar Bath:** This helps relieve sore muscles, itchy skin, and sunburn. Vinegar helps draw pollutants out of the body. It is an acid medium and contains alpha hydroxy acids. It is also mildly antiseptic, antifungal, and naturally deodorizing. You can even infuse therapeutic herbs into the vinegar to make an herbal vinegar. Add 1/4 to 1 cup apple cider vinegar to your bath herbs and let it steep for two weeks to a month. Strain the herbs out before using and rebottle the vinegar. Herbs to steep into the vinegar might include: calendula, chamomile, lavender, lemon balm, peppermint, spearmint, rose petals, sage, and scented geraniums.

- **Athlete's Bath:** Use these ingredients to relax sore aching muscles: bay leaf, Epsom salts, eucalyptus leaves, gingerroot, juniper berries, lavender flowers, marjoram herb, mustard seed powder, rosemary leaves, or sage herb.

- **Baking Soda Bath:** This alkalinizing and detoxifying bath can help calm allergic reactions, chicken pox, eczema, hives, itchy skin, insect bites, poison ivy, sunburn, and fungal infections. Baking soda baths also aid weight loss. Use one pound of baking soda per bath.

- **Blemished Skin Bath:** Include these skin clearing ingredients in your bath: apple cider vinegar, lavender, lemon peel, or tea tree oil.

- **Brain Stimulating Bath:** These herbs help relax the body but invigorate the mind: grapefruit peel, lemon peel, orange peel, peppermint leaves, pine needles, or tangerine peel.

- **Cold and Flu Bath:** Try these bath additions when you want to soothe deep muscle aches that often accompany viral infections: Epsom salts, gingerroot, marjoram, mustard seed powder, pine needles, or thyme leaves.

- **Cornstarch:** Added to a bath, cornstarch is softening and calms itchy skin. Use it for skin irritations or diaper rash. Don't use cornstarch if you are dealing with yeast infections.

- **Detox Bath:** Use these cleansing herbs in the bath when you know it's time to change your lifestyle and help your body get rid of environmental pollutants and internal toxins and cleanse your lymphatic system: apple cider vinegar, cypress essential oil, Epsom salts, gingerroot, grapefruit, juniper, lavender flowers, lemon peel, rosemary leaves, sage leaves, sea vegetables (purchase these dried from natural food stores unless you live close to the ocean), or tea tree essential oil.

- **Dry Skin Bath:** Herbs can have a soothing, lubricating effect externally. Moisturize with calendula flowers, chamomile flowers, comfrey leaves, elder flowers, fennel seed, jasmine flowers, lavender flowers, rolled oats, rosebuds, or violet leaves. Consider mixing up a rich bath oil made with 1/2 cup each of the following: avocado oil, safflower oil, sunflower oil, and almond oil; then add 1/2 ounce of pure lavender oil. Shake the oils together and add 2 tablespoons to your bath. Adding oil to a tub can cause slippery conditions, so be sure to have a shower mat.

- **Empowerment Bath:** Add quartz crystals to your bath (make sure they are large enough so they don't go down the drain) for their healing and energy clearing properties.

- **Energizing Bath:** Enliven your spirits with stimulating bergamot, coriander, cypress, eucalyptus leaves, grapefruit peel, juniper berry, lemon peel, lime peel, orange peel, peppermint leaves, pine needles, or rosemary leaves. A folk remedy to perk you up is to eat a crisp sour apple while in a tepid bath.

- **Epsom Salts Bath:** This bath cleanses the lymphatic channels, relaxes sore muscles, softens the skin, and is detoxifying after bodywork. Epsom salts help draw out drugs, chemicals, and pollutants from the body. People with diabetes, hypertension, or heart disease should rinse off well after bathing with Epsom salts.

- **Flower Essence Bath:** Bach Flower Essences and Rescue Remedy can be added to the bath for emotional health and balance. Simply add two drops to a filled tub.

- **Flower Power Bath:** Float fresh flowers or orange or lemon peels in the bathwater. Flower suggestions include lilacs, dandelions, daisies, honeysuckle, jasmine, camellia, or lavender. Trim aromatic leaves (mint, lemon balm, and so forth) and put them into the bath.

- **Hot Weather Bath:** Beat the heat with herbs that refresh and revitalize. Cool off with lemon peel and peppermint leaves. You can even throw in a few lemon halves that you have left over after making fresh lemonade.

- **Itchy Skin Bath:** To calm itchy skin caused by insect bites, chicken pox, or poison ivy, bathe with apple cider vinegar, baking soda, chickweed herb, lavender flowers, powdered rolled oats, red clover blossoms, or violet leaf. Essential oils to use in an itchy-skin bath include cedarwood, Roman chamomile, lavender, peppermint, or sandalwood.

- **Kid's Bath:** Make bath time more fun with flowers and fragrance. Try hibiscus flowers (they will turn the bathwater pink), lavender flowers, blue malva flowers (they will turn the bathwater purple), orange flowers, or rosebuds.

- **Lover's Bath:** Stimulate your senses with herbs that have long been considered passion potions. Use cardamom pods, cinnamon bark pieces, jasmine flowers, rosebuds, ylang-ylang flowers, or sandalwood (use sandalwood only if it has been ethically harvested, as sandalwood is rare in the wild). You can also try pure vanilla extract. Add three tablespoons of pure extract to put you in the mood for love.

- **Mood-Lifting Happy Bath:** Add tangerine peels or any other citrus peels to the bathwater. Why not slowly and sensuously enjoy a piece of fruit in the bath as you soak with the peel (providing you are not allergic to citrus fruits). Essential oils to use include bergamot, clary sage, frankincense, geranium, jasmine, mandarin, melissa (lemon balm), or palmarosa.

- **Mud Bath:** These are very detoxifying and antibacterial. They are useful for infections, pain, swelling, gout, arthritis, kidney failure, cancer, lupus, eczema, and poison ivy. Mud baths are easy to do at a spa that provides this service.

- **Oatmeal Bath:** This calms irritated skin, poison ivy, dermatitis, high blood pressure, and stress. It is very simple to whiz rolled oats in the blender to make a bath powder. Alternatively, tie 1/2 cup rolled oats into a bath bag.

- **Oily Skin Bath:** Help balance oil production with basil leaf, lemon peel, or apple cider vinegar.

- **Premenstrual Bath:** Calm cramps and emotional upheaval with nature's bounty of chamomile flowers, clary sage flowers, or lavender flowers.

- **Rejuvenative Bath:** Many herbs contain natural antioxidant properties that can help deter cellular damage. Consider using lavender flowers, rosemary leaves, or ylang-ylang flowers.

- **Relaxing Bath:** Take the edge off a stressful day with calming botanicals such as catnip herb, chamomile flowers, clary sage flowers, hops strobiles, jasmine flowers, lavender flowers, linden flowers, neroli flowers, or rosebuds.

- **Salt Bath:** Herbalist and teacher William LeSassier always said salt and baking soda baths help clean the health aura. Salt helps to soften the skin and has been used to treat burns. Salt baths are good after bodywork and for eczema, psoriasis, rashes, and sore muscles. Baking soda mixed with salt is suggested after exposure to radiation. Use 1/2 to 2 cups of sea salt. People with insulin dependent diabetes, serious heart disease, and open sores should avoid salt baths. Salt can sting on an open cut!

- **Seaweed Bath:** This is excellent after bodywork and for glandular imbalances and helping to promote weight loss. It is also good when you want to pretend you're a mermaid. Use seaweed baths to help draw environmental pollutants from the body, including radiation. Sea vegetables are rejuvenative and soothe sunburn. Any edible sea vegetable can be used.

- **Sensitive Skin Bath:** Almost any skin type can tolerate and benefit from lavender, lemon verbena, linden flower, rose petals, and spearmint.

- **Sunburn Bath:** Adding black tea or apple cider vinegar to a cool bath eases burns.

- **Weight-Loss Bath:** These herbs stimulate circulation and have traditionally been used to aid weight loss: burdock root, fennel seed, juniper berry, kelp, lemon peel, orange peel, parsley leaf, peppermint leaf, rosemary leaf, and sea vegetables. Use an herb-filled cloth to gently scrub parts of your body that need to be slenderized.

When bathing, for at least a moment, submerge the crown of your head or float with the back of your head and crown tilted back to complete the circuit (unless you simply can't get your hair wet). It is most relaxing.

When you are done bathing, visualize the tension draining out of you, as the water runs out of the tub, and being soothed by the warm water and Earth Mother. Rise carefully from the bath to avoid light-headedness. Follow the bath with a cool rinse, if desired.

You can start with cool temperatures and gradually build up your tolerance. Traditional hydrotherapy suggests not toweling off but rinsing with cool water and then putting on your clothes. This helps dry skin retain moisture and strengthens the immune system.

Hot showers are relaxing and improve circulation; they are more deeply penetrating than cold showers. Hot showers stimulate the blood's flow to the surface of the skin, imparting a rosy glow. Cold showers contract the blood vessels and are energizing. Long cold showers help desensitize a person to pain. Showers can also be directed to a certain part of the body to center energy and increase blood flow where it may be needed, such as concentrating the spray on the perineum for prostate problems. Turn your soles upward and spray your feet for a reflexology treatment. Concentrating the spray on the abdomen can help constipation. Directing the spray on the chest can increase respiration and help breathing conditions, such as asthma, with dramatic results. Alternate hot and cold showers to relieve minor aches and pains, chronic back pain, and stiff joints.

The way to health is to have an aromatic bath and a scented massage every day.

—HIPPOCRATES

A few drops of lavender or tea tree essential oil can be added to a sponge when giving a sponge bath.

Getting clean is only part of the therapy. Bathe your body. Soothe your soul. Appreciate the beautiful blessings of water!

Bath Salts

It's easy to create your own bath salts with this simple mixture. Using a seashell as a scoop makes a delightful gift addition. Add one handful per filled bath.

1 cup sea salt
1 cup baking soda
1 cup Epsom salts
1 teaspoon essential oil(s) of your choice

Combine the sea salt, baking soda, and Epsom salts in a bowl. Add the essential oil and mix well. Store in a glass jar.

Bath Fizz

Watch this whiz and fizz!

1 cup baking soda
3 tablespoons citric acid
7 drops essential oil of your choice

Combine all of the ingredients. Add about three heaping tablespoons of the mixture per bath.

Hot Springs and Spas

Hot springs open the pores and nourish our skin with minerals. In earlier times, spas offered massage, exercise, dance, music, and theater as part of the therapy. In Germany, entire towns were dedicated as health spas, indicated by the word *bad*, meaning "bath" or "spa." Mud baths are drawing and cleansing, but they also can be drying and must be rinsed well so the mud doesn't clog the pores. Thalassotherapy (*thalassa* means "sea" in Greek) incorporates using seawater and plants as therapy. It is also sometimes referred to as marinetherapy in North America and balneotherapy in Europe. Our plasma (the liquid part of the blood) is very similar to the mineral content of the sea. The sea is our true ancestral home, and seawater contains all the elements needed for cellular function. Bathe in the ocean when you can.

Saunas

Sweat is about 98 percent water and 2 percent solids. Sweat lodges were used in America, Europe, Asia, and Africa as a way of cleansing the body and soul. Saunas can be overly drying; to make them less so, pour water over the rocks (be aware that this will temporarily increase the temperature). Saunas help relax muscle spasms, relieve arthritis, aid in the elimination of waste materials (including lactic acid), help weight loss, open the respiratory passages, clean and open the pores of the skin, increase circulation, relax tight muscles, and reduce anxiety and stress. They can also help release stuck emotions and heal trauma.

Share water, Brother.

—VALENTINE MICHAEL SMITH, *STRANGER IN A STRANGE LAND*, BY ROBERT A. HEINLEIN

Avoid eating a heavy meal one to two hours prior to using a sauna. Clean your skin well first. It is best to enter the sauna with dry skin. Remove any jewelry and eyeglasses, including contact lenses, as they can get too dry and irritate the eyes. Protect delicate skin by covering your face with a wet towel or cloth, and limit sauna time to no longer than ten to twelve minutes. Praying, meditating, or light exercise are encouraged while in the sauna.

Skin temperatures may rise to as high as 104 degrees in less than five minutes. As a reaction, sweating is induced, which cools the skin. Surface blood vessels enlarge, allowing more nourishment for the cells of the skin. Dry heat is especially beneficial for acne and other skin disorders. Saunas are more drawing than steam baths. Splashing water on the rocks creates negative ions and helps keep the capillaries on sensitive skin from breaking.

To add a freshening aroma to your sauna, combine 10–15 drops essential oil to 16 ounces water. Throw a bit at a time onto the sauna rocks. Never put undiluted oils on sauna heat as it can cause an explosion. Eucalyptus, fir, and tea tree are good essential oils for saunas.

When relaxing in the sauna, it is beneficial to move back and forth between elevations and to elevate your legs. After several minutes of being in there, dry brush skin massage can be practiced. Drink lots of fluids and even diaphoretic herbal teas. Up to half a gallon of water can be lost as the body perspires.

- Take a cold shower between sauna visits. Cold plunges are also often taken as the finale.
- Taking drugs or medications before a sauna can intensify the effects of both and should be preceded with extreme caution, if used at all. If anything becomes excessively uncomfortable, stop.
- A suggested sauna routine is to take a warm shower for two minutes, followed by a ten-minute sauna. Then do a one-minute cold plunge or short swim, or throw snow on yourself. Follow this with a second ten-minute sauna, a cold plunge for one minute, another ten-minute sauna, a one-minute cold treatment, and end with a cool shower and gentle scrubbing.
- A cold plunge after a sauna increases adrenal activity and can be very psychedelic. Dry saunas can be dehydrating; drink plenty of liquid.

THE BEAUTIFUL PLEASURES OF MASSAGE

The sensation of touch corresponds to our earliest memories of being cared for in our mother's arms. Massage is one of the most ancient forms of health and beauty care. It helps move blocked energy in the body, improves circulation, stimulates all the meridians, relieves muscle tension, improves posture, decreases stress, and even elevates mood. Through the time-tested actions of stroking, kneading, and pressing, heart rate is improved, blood pressure is reduced, and breathing and digestion are enhanced. Occasional massages are a wonderful way to turn inward, honor and nurture yourself, and enhance a more intimate connection with your body. Taking time out occasionally for a good massage can be relaxing, aligning, and moisturizing. When applying lotions in cold weather or wanting to rub some on your beloved, to avoid shocking cold jolts, put the bottle of lotion in a cup of hot water for a few minutes before applying. Avoid deep direct massage during infection, after recent surgery, or when skin is infected or inflamed, and be extra careful during pregnancy.

Ask your friends and colleagues for their recommendations for a good massage therapist in your area. You may want to try several different styles of massage and see which one suits you best. You might not always have time to receive a full body massage, but scalp, face, hand, foot, and back rubs can be relished and help you glow! I like to schedule massages at the end of the day, so I don't have to rush back to work and can enjoy the afterglow for the rest of the day.

Massage is usually given on a professional massage table, but it can be done on a sheet on the floor. Often the room is warm and softly lit. Good massage therapists might wash their hands in hot water before touching you, or rub them together to increase warmth.

The lightest and most pleasant base oils for massage are grapeseed, sunflower, and safflower. My favorite massage oils are raw coconut oil and extra-virgin olive oil. Avoid oils that are heavy, possibly allergenic, and odiferous, such as peanut or corn oil. Massage oil can go rancid, so it is best to keep most of it in the refrigerator, leaving out just enough for a few days. The bottle of massage oil can be warmed by placing it in a cup of hot water for a few minutes. You most likely won't want oil used on your scalp, or your hair will look oily and heavy.

Many massage therapists encourage feedback. You can ask for harder, softer, deeper, or slower, but don't spoil the experience by talking too much and being in your head or you'll miss out on the true massage experience.

There are many types of massage to choose from. Different types may be beneficial at various times in your life. A great Web site that describes hundreds of massage types is www.massagetherapy.com. Here are just a few types of massage techniques and therapies:

- **Acupressure**, also known as shiatsu, uses finger pressure rather than needles to stimulate various acupuncture points. It also incorporates stretching and movement.
- **Alexander Technique** emphasizes changing our habitual ways of moving our head, neck, and torso, and focuses on each body part's relationship with gravity.
- **Aston-Patterning** combines movement, bodywork, ergonomics, and fitness training to help us become aware of stressful movement habits. It uses deep tissue manipulation, muscle direction and lubrication, and smoothing the fascia.
- **Berrywork** uses corrective stretches that involve the cartilage, fascia, and joints.
- **Cranial sacral therapy** improves the pulsation of cerebral spinal fluids and helps release blockages with very tiny movements.
- **Deep tissue work** uses fingers, elbows, forearms, and even toes to apply pressure to soften and lengthen the body's connective fibers.
- **Feldenkrais Method** helps improve the way the body organizes itself to improve structure and alignment.
- **Hellerwork** incorporates deep tissue work that affects the musculature and nervous system, movement reeducation, and observation of how emotions affect the body.

- **Integrative Massage** moves energy from the head out through the hands and feet.
- **Jin shin jitsu** is gentle and noninvasive; clients remain fully clothed. The practitioner attunes to the body's pulses and helps release blockages.
- **LaStone Therapy** uses a variety of rocks that range in temperature from 0 to 140 degrees to promote health and relaxation and a connection to the earth's energies.
- **Lomilomi** uses large broad movements and originated in Hawaii.
- **Lymphatic drainage massage** helps improve lymphatic drainage when the trained practitioner palpates the flow of lymph movement.
- **Myofascial release** applies pressure and movement into the fascial system to allow for the release of emotions and patterns that no longer serve the body's highest potential.
- **Polarity Therapy** helps balance the electromagnetic currents of the body. Gentle manual manipulation is one method of opening the blockages, along with diet, stretching, and emotional release.
- **Postural Integration** uses deep tissue manipulation and deep breathing to release blocked energy and improve posture.
- **Reflexology**, also known as zone therapy, does massage mostly on the feet and hands to improve the flow of energy throughout the body's meridians.
- **Rolfing** is a deep tissue technique that restructures the body. It can increase flexibility, lengthen the muscles, and release emotional blockages.
- **Russian massage** uses basic massage strokes and maximizes the comfort of the client.
- **Swedish massage** focuses on strokes that go toward the heart and improve circulation. Swedish massage is used to relieve muscle spasms and tension, reduce lactic acid, and improve mobility.
- **Trager work** consists of gentle, simple exercises such as light rocking or shaking to help the client overcome resistance and become more relaxed.
- **Watsu** is a delightful therapy that involves being massaged while you are submerged in water. We lose about 90 percent of our body weight when underwater, which allows the therapist to do some deep and effective work.

The Crane

The Crane is a Taoist exercise that is a type of self-massage that improves digestion, sleep, reduces mental chatter, and helps you have a flatter tummy.

1. Lie down flat on your back. Relax and place the palm of your dominant hand on your navel. Just rub clockwise from the center making small circles that gradually expand, covering a larger area of the belly.
2. Reverse hands and directions, rubbing counterclockwise in smaller and smaller circles till you reach the navel's center. Visualize a warm flow of energy moving from your hand into your center and the organs within. Concentrate and be present.

During the first portion of the exercise you are massaging the organs of digestion and elimination. Fatty accumulations are dispersed and moved into the channels of elimination. When you go clockwise, bowel action is improved. Being overweight and constipated often go hand in hand. Rubbing counterclockwise helps move water from the small intestines to the kidneys. Repeat this exercise first thing in the morning before getting up and last thing at night when lying down.

Massaging the Face

Facial massage improves blood circulation and collagen production, can help release stored tensions, and can help prevent wrinkles. Daily facial massage can help dull-looking skin to become more vibrant, bright, and relaxed. After a facial massage, we appear more youthful and feel supercharged. Just as physical exercise keeps the body fit, facial exercises can help firm, lift, and tonify the face without the risks, expense, and other problems of surgery. There are fifteen facial muscles, and exercising any of them affects the others to some degree. Facial exercises can be done before bed, while you watch TV or allow your conditioner to soak in, or whenever you are feeling stressed.

Some beauty authorities feel that facial massage and exercises are not helpful; they do not believe that loss of muscle tone is a big factor in sagging skin and that lines caused by facial movement are not likely to be helped. In addition, they contend that anything that moves the skin can contribute to loss of elasticity and create even more wrinkling. You will have to decide for yourself. I have found that doing facial massage releases tension and improves my looks. If you choose to do facial exercises, do so with well-moisturized skin.

When cleansing, scrubbing, toning, and moisturizing, some simple facial massage techniques can be employed while you are applying the products of your choice; they can improve circulation and make your beauty ritual more intentional. Try these techniques in front of a mirror the first few times to make them easier. Learning these techniques until they become second nature will serve you well!

Facial Massage #1

This helps smooth lines on the forehead.

1. Massage small circles across your forehead. Begin at your right temple and move across to the left.
2. Using a crisscross pattern, massage across your forehead, working from left to right.
3. Without lifting your fingers, use smooth even movements to do effleurage (soothing, rhythmic stroking) across your forehead.
4. Repeat each step seven times.

Facial Massage #2

This helps correct sagging eye muscles and improves skin tone.

1. Make a large oval O with your mouth, pulling your upper lip over your teeth.
2. Without moving your mouth, smile. This will cause your upper cheeks to lift while your eyes are squeezed shut.
3. While holding this position, use the fingertips of both hands to make complete circles around your eyes, always beginning at the inner corner, over your eyebrows, to the outer corners, then under your eyes (including your upper cheeks), making a full circle. Do this about five times or while slowly counting to ten.

Facial Massage #3

This improves circulation to the nose.

1. Lightly massage your nose with downward strokes.
2. Massage down your nose with small circular strokes, starting at the top of the nose and moving downward.
3. Repeat seven times. End by massaging the tip of your nose and pressing it in and up. Hold for a count of seven.

Facial Massage #4

This keeps the lower portion of the face firm and helps prevent and correct double chins and jowls.

1. Roll your lips inward over your lower and upper teeth, leaving approximately one-half inch between your lips. Smile as wide as possible with your lower jaw, as if grinning up to your ears. Avoid moving the rest of your face.

2. While holding this position, massage your lower face in small outward circles, beginning at the tip of your chin, moving toward your ears, then moving back down again, while slowly counting to ten.
3. Still holding the position, make a full circle around your mouth seven times using your fingertips from both hands; then do seven circles in the opposite direction.

Facial Massage #5

This will improve droopy corners of your mouth.

1. Smile with your mouth closed.
2. Curl your lips exaggeratedly upward.

Facial Massage #6

Use this technique to smooth upper lip lines, decrease furrows from your mouth to the corners of your chin, firm and fill out your lips, and strengthen the muscles that surround your mouth.

1. With your lips together in a straight line, make a slight smile.
2. While counting to ten, massage tiny outward circles around your mouth using the index fingers of both hands.
3. Continue squeezing the muscles of your lips harder until a tingling sensation is felt around your mouth. Then make a small puckered O shape with your mouth, as if you were about to kiss and smile slightly.
4. Massage tiny outward circles all the way around your mouth as you slowly count to ten.
5. Using a light touch, make a circle around your eye area, beginning at the inner corner of each eye and moving up to the brows and back to each eye corner. Repeat seven times.

Facial Massage #7

This helps firm and smooth the neck.

1. With your thumb directly beneath your chin, curl your tongue to the back of your mouth till you can feel the muscle that is directly under your chin protrude. Then release your thumb, still keeping your tongue in its curled place.
2. Stretch your neck as far left as possible, chin pointing upward, and slowly rotate to the right. With the fingers of both hands, beginning at the base of your neck, massage in long, vigorous, upward strokes toward the jawbone as you move your neck in a semicircle from left to right. Continue for a slow count of ten.

Facial Acupressure

According to Asian tradition, the face is a map of the body, just as are the feet, eyes, and hands. On the next page is a chart that shows which part of the face corresponds to the body's inner workings. For example, where we break out may be an indication of what is going on inside our body.

Facial acupressure is a great way to de-stress your face and improve circulation, thus encouraging a more beautiful visage.

Acupressure Face-Lift

Acupressure facial massage presses tsubos, or special points. This helps relax the face, and improve circulation, and move stagnancy, where lines and wrinkles are most likely to form. This is done with your knuckle or thumbs or the end of a rounded makeup brush, not needles. The best time to practice Acupressure Face-Lift is after cleansing your skin. Practice this at least twice a week.

1. Apply serum or moisturizer to your face. Press slowly and firmly, pressing inward against the bone, not downward or upward. Simply press, using moderate pressure, for about ten seconds, using a circular clockwise motion. Making small circles while maintaining pressure and moving the skin over the bone is ideal. Hold for seven seconds.
2. Release and repeat. Using this technique, press each of the points depicted on page 92. Practice nightly after cleansing. You can even do a facial steam first. This massage can be practiced while you are in the bath. Avoid pulling and tugging on your skin. Be sure to use a quality moisturizer.

Massage Oil

It is easy to make your own massage oil. I like to use a plastic bottle with a squeeze top so that if it falls on the floor during a massage, I don't have a disaster to deal with. Essential oils give massage oil a wonderful and therapeutic aroma. Try lavender, rosemary, birch, juniper, or any other essential oil you prefer.

4 ounces carrier oil (such as coconut, grapeseed, sesame, or almond oil)

40 drops essential oil of your choice

Pour the carrier oil into a clean, dry bottle. Add the essential oil and shake well. Store your oil in a cool, dark place.

Facial Diagnosis Chart

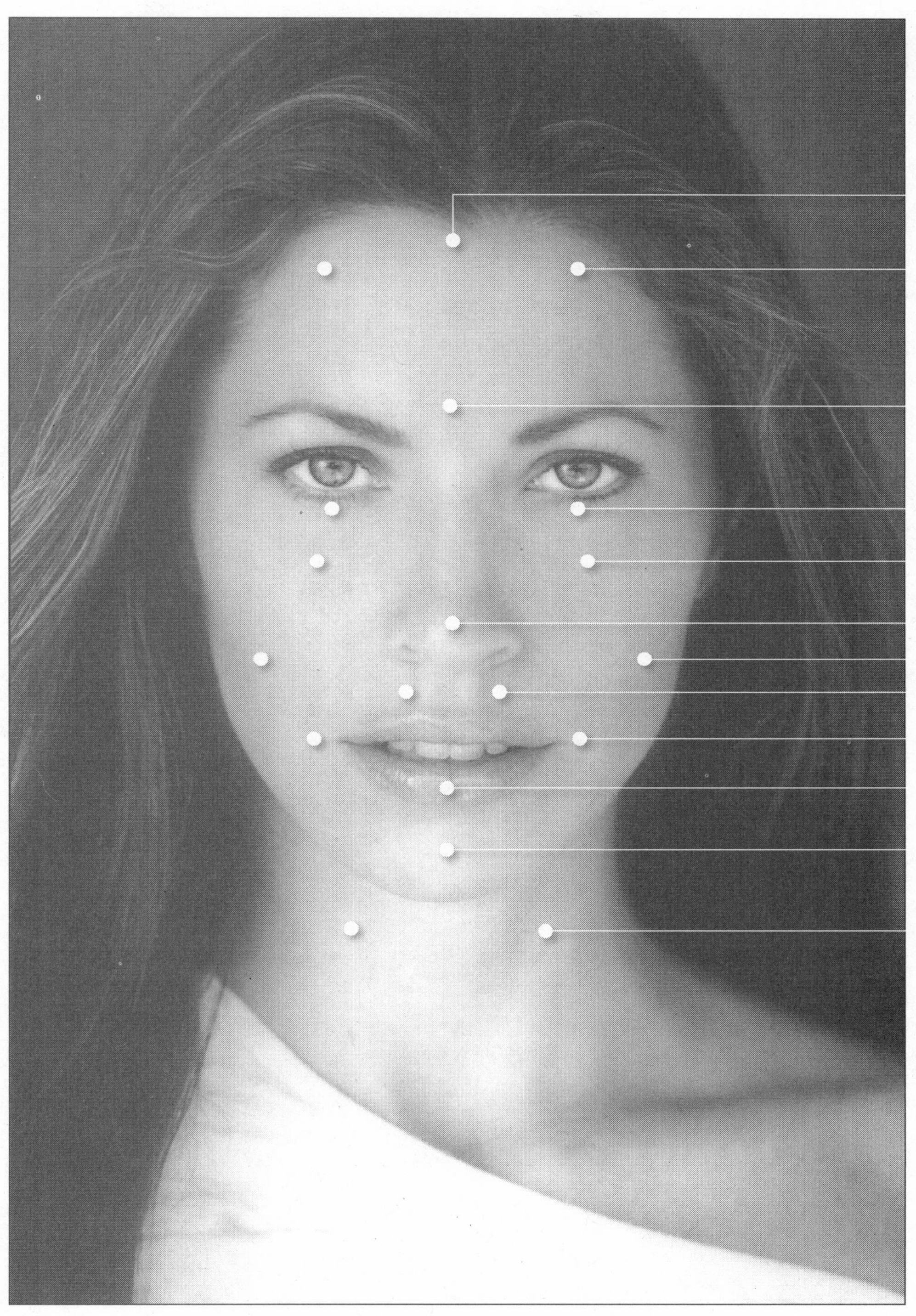

Facial Acupressure Chart

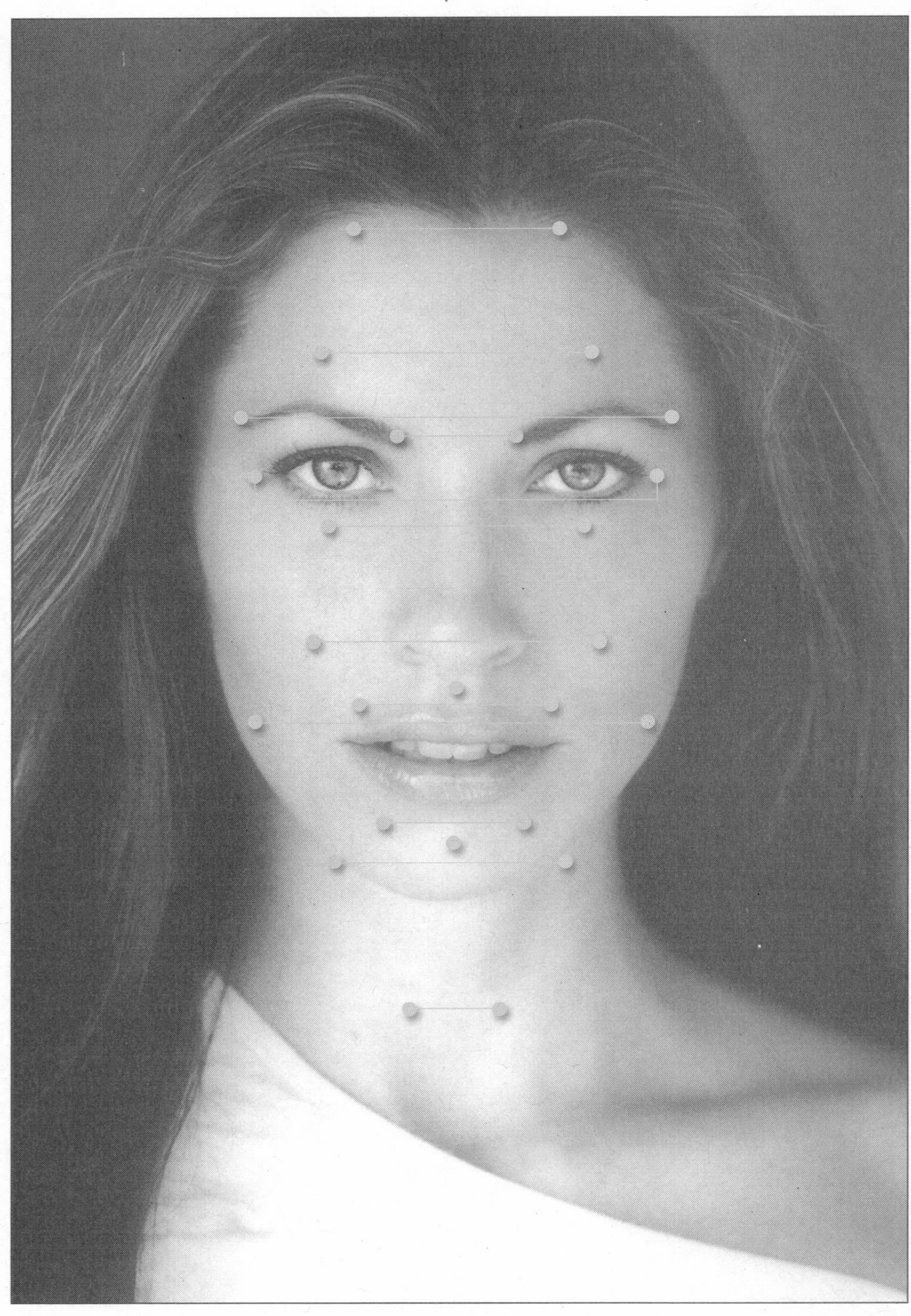

AROMATHERAPY ADDITIONS FOR CARRIER OIL

- **Cold and Flu Massage:** eucalyptus, lavender, and pine.
- **Improve Your Mood Blend:** basil, geranium, lemon, and peppermint.
- **Invigorating Massage:** geranium, lemon, lime, and peppermint or spearmint.
- **Rejuvenative Massage:** frankincense, jasmine, melissa, patchouli, and/or rose.
- **Relaxing Massage:** chamomile, lavender, sandalwood, and hops.
- **Sensual Massage:** cardamom, jasmine, neroli, patchouli, rose, tuberose, vanilla, or ylang-ylang.
- **Sore Muscles Massage:** birch, fir, juniper, and/or rosemary.
- **Weight-Loss Massage:** fennel seed, juniper, or lemon.

Sports Muscle Oil

Apply this after exertion to relax sore muscles.

1/2 cup coconut oil
15 drops peppermint essential oil
15 drops rosemary essential oil
5 drops ginger essential oil
5 drops eucalyptus essential oil

Combine all the ingredients in a wide-mouth jar. Apply as needed, but avoid mucous membranes.

Warming Body Oil

Feel the warming *chi* moving through your being.

1/2 cup coconut oil
30 drops juniper essential oil
5 drops ginger essential oil
5 drops rosemary essential oil

Combine all the ingredients in a clean eight-ounce squeeze bottle.

CHAPTER 3

Beautiful Body by Nature

BEAUTIFUL HAIR

Hair, often referred to as our crowning glory, can add to our beauty and individuality. Hair can protect the head from sun or excessive cold and shield us from injury. Some people consider hair to be like an antenna, connecting us to universal energies.

Hair can also be thought of like a blade of grass. Each hair has its own life cycle. It will grow strong and healthy, providing the soil is rich. Poor nutrition, hormonal changes, negative emotions such as envy and hatred, overexposure to the sun, chemicals, chlorinated water and swimming pools, pollutants, and alcohol consumption can all impair hair health. Taking better care of your health will eventually improve your hair, but it may take several months for the benefits to show, since hair grows slowly. In Asian medicine, the health of the hair is a reflection of the strength of the kidneys and blood.

Anatomy of Hair

Healthy hair is strong, slightly oily, and self-renewing. Trichology is the science and study of hair, including the physical, emotional, and environmental aspects of the hair and scalp.

Since hair doesn't contain any nerves, it is considered nonliving tissue. The portion that is living is below the scalp.

Hair is comprised of 95–97 percent protein and 3 percent moisture. One of the main components of hair is the fibrous protein keratin, which is made of eighteen amino acids. Keratin is arranged in a double helix formation and also occurs in human nails as well as animals' claws, horns, feathers, and fur. Keratin fibers are held together by several polypeptide bonds. The strongest is from the sulfur-containing amino acid cystine. Hair, in general, is a high-nitrogen-containing substance. Light-colored hair contains less hydrogen and carbon than brunette hair, but more oxygen and sulfur.

The cortex is made of millions of hard, parallel protein fibers and is held together by various bonds, protected by the cuticle. It is responsible for about 90 percent of the hair's molecular weight and determines its texture. The cuticle is an outer protective layer composed of overlapping scales or cells, similar to the shingles on a roof or a coat of armor, that protects against environmental and self-induced hair stresses. The cuticle has an inner and outer coat and surrounds a mass of spindle-shaped cells called the paracortex and orthocortex. It is the cuticle that gives the hair its color, elasticity, and strength. When the cuticles neatly overlap and lie flat, the hair looks shiny and soft. If the cuticle becomes broken (either chemically or physically), the hair will tangle easily and appear dull and brittle.

Mom was right. We lose up to 35 percent of our body's heat through our head. Wearing a hat will keep you warmer.

Each hair has a medulla, or thin, hollow inner core of transparent polygon-shaped cells made of fat granules, pigment, and air spaces; the medulla may be missing in very fine hair.

Hair grows out of the scalp, and it is the skin that contains the hair root, erector pili muscle, sebaceous glands, hair shaft, and blood vessels. It is the erector pili muscle that determines the direction in which the hair grows.

At the hair follicle's base is the papilla, or "root," through which oxygenated blood nourishes the hair via the capillaries. It is also here that the sebaceous glands make the oily substance sebum. It is the follicle's shape that determines whether our hair will be straight or curly. When observed in a cross section, straight hair is round, wavy hair oval shaped, and curly hair is more kidney shaped. Straight hair has roots that produce the same number of keratin cells all around the hair follicle. With curly hair, the number of keratin cells is uneven.

The average scalp has about 100,000 hairs. A single strand of hair can last from two to four years. Hair usually grows one-half inch per month. Most hair tends to be thicker in the summer and fall out more in autumn. It is normal to lose between fifty and one hundred and fifty hairs a day. This is not a problem unless we lose more than is replaced. Women's hair tends to grow faster than men's. Hair grows the fastest when we are between age fifteen and thirty. After age fifty, hair growth will slow down somewhat. In an average lifetime, hair will grow about twenty-five feet. When hair grows, new cells overlap the older cells.

Hair Nutrition

Foods for healthy hair include almonds, blackberries, papayas, plums, dark green leafy vegetables, celery, green beans, sweet potatoes, pumpkin, sesame and sunflower seeds, barley, buckwheat, millet, oats (good for hair loss due to illness), rice, rye, and yogurt. Eating sea vegetables is said to keep hair healthy and dark, especially arame, hijiki, kombu, and wakame. Also beneficial for the hair are the sulfur-rich vegetables garlic and onions. Since hair is made of protein, make sure you are getting adequate supplies. My favorite protein sources are raw nuts, raw seeds, sun-cured olives, spirulina, sunflower sprouts, avocado, and green leafy vegetables.

Vegetable juices that promote healthy hair include beet, carrot, cucumber, spinach, and onion. Always dilute vegetable juices 50 percent with water, as they are very concentrated.

Teas to drink for healthy hair include alfalfa, burdock root, ho shou wu, horsetail, nettle, and oat straw.

If you are eating a diet high in raw food, you probably won't need vitamin supplements. However, people are on different paths at different times in life, and natural food stores do carry vitamin blends specifically for healthy hair. The following are some possible ingredients in these blends and how they can help your hair.

Vitamin A deficiency can lead to a dry, flaky scalp as well as hair loss. Vitamin B complex helps relieve stress, curb hair loss, and helps regulate oil production. Especially important are PABA (para-amino benzoic acid) and inositol (part of the B complex), which help protect the hair follicles. PABA, biotin, folic acid, and pantothenic acid, all part of the B-complex vitamins, help protect hair color. Vitamin C enhances circulation to the scalp, and a lack of it may make hair more likely to break. Vitamin E increases the body's utilization of oxygen and thus improves circulation to the scalp. Include foods with essential fatty acids in your diet, such as flaxseed oil, to help balance both dry and oily scalp. Silica helps nourish hair as well as skin and nails. Hair contains a high concentration of zinc; therefore supplementing with zinc can also be helpful. Cysteine is a component of hair that promotes the formation of keratin and collagen.

When hair is in good health, it should be elastic enough to stretch 30 percent beyond its resting range and then spring back to its original size and shape. Hair has the ability to absorb up to 50 percent its weight in water. When hair is "normal," its porosity can vary from slightly to extremely porous. The hair strand can swell to 120 percent of its regular diameter. One way to test porosity is to take one hair from the top of your head, each side, and the back. Drop them into a bowl of water. You'll know your hair is very porous if it sinks within ten seconds. Such hair is fragile, and must be especially well conditioned.

Hair Health

Many hair concerns are really due to what is going on in the scalp, where the hair is housed. Smoking and lack of exercise can impair circulation to the scalp.

Scalp massages are wonderfully relaxing, promote hair beauty, help prevent hair loss, stimulate the sebaceous glands, and improve circulation. You can do a scalp massage before washing your hair. It is also good to do in the morning and evening with just three to four drops of rosemary essential oil. Do small circular motions, using only the pads of your fingers, for one minute in each area of your scalp. Work from your hairline to the sides, then over the crown to the base of your neck, the way the blood flows to the heart. Bending your head forward while doing the scalp massage is especially beneficial.

Another scalp treat is to gently knock on the skull (without any oils) using the knuckles of both hands; continue until you feel like stopping. You can also take a large handful of hair and gently tug on it to strengthen the hair and scalp.

Hair Brushing

Many people spend more time on their hair than on any other body part. Brushing the hair helps distribute the scalp's oils to the full length of the hair and increases circulation to the scalp. Brushing gives hair fullness and helps the hair create a soft halo around the face. Brushing is especially important for long hair. It is good to brush hair before washing it.

Use a brush with natural bristles, as it will absorb the hair's natural oils so they can be better distributed. Natural bristles also do a better job of removing dirt and dust. Plastic bristles, unlike natural bristles, don't distribute or absorb oil and are more likely to create static.

Start brushing at the ends of your hair and work up, brushing a few inches higher after every few strokes. If you are not used to brushing one hundred strokes, start with a lower number and gradually work up. Hold your hair while brushing it to avoid tugging at your scalp. To give hair more body, brush it while bending over. Avoid brushing your hair when it is wet, as then it will have weaker hydrogen bonds and be more likely to break; it is okay to comb your hair during conditioning. Many people find it relaxing to brush their hair before bed.

Every time you wash your hairbrush, ideally every couple of weeks, you can soak it in soapy tepid water; then rinse it well and dry it with the bristles facing downward on clean, dry towels. Apply one or two drops of essential oil (my favorite is rosemary) directly to your brush, if desired.

Hair Care Tips

- Chemical processes, such as coloring and perms, can dry the hair when used repeatedly. Perms break down the inner structure of the hair, causing it to become misshapen. Perms alter the hair's natural keratin and break down the sulfur bonds of the hair.
- Rubber bands damage hair by causing breakage when they are removed. It is better to use coated hair ties or metal-free elastic bands, if needed, as the metal portion tends to tangle and break the hair.
- Avoid wearing tight barrettes, clips, or ties to bed. Hair needs to "breathe," so it is best to avoid wearing tight hats, bands, and wigs that prevent circulation to the scalp. Tight hairstyles worn over extended periods, such as ponytails and braids, can contribute to hair loss or breakage. Wear your hair loose when possible to avoid pulling at the scalp.
- Avoid excessive heat, such as sitting close to a fire or being in the sun without a hat. After swimming in a pool or ocean, be sure to rinse your hair well.
- On windy days (or when riding in a convertible), tie your hair to keep it from getting overly tangled.
- Minimize the use of blow-dryers, electric curling implements (hot rollers and curling irons), and chlorinated swimming pools. If you must blow-dry your hair, wait till your hair is almost dry rather than dripping wet to save energy and preserve your hair. Keep the dryer on a low or cool setting. Hold it at least six inches away from your hair, and keep it moving. A leave-in conditioner will also help protect hair from the consequences of blow-drying. I prefer to dry my hair in the sun or allow it to air-dry by letting the breezes blow through it.

Hair Washing

Hair, ideally, should not be washed every day. Oily hair can be washed every other day. Less oily hair can get by with a washing twice a week.

Overwashing the hair tends to make it oilier, as the sebaceous glands become stimulated to produce more oil to compensate. Before shampooing, brush or comb hair with a wide-tooth comb, starting at the bottom of the hair.

Choose shampoos that are made with olive, coconut, or palm oil. Shampoos that are labeled "pH balanced" have the same level of acidity as hair. Alkaline shampoos can be overly drying. Check out the Resources section (page 229) for quality, effective, natural-as-possible products. Read the instructions on the shampoo and conditioner bottles. Hair care experts say it is good to switch shampoo and conditioner brands to avoid a buildup of residue. Before adding shampoo, rinse hair with warm water to prewash it, and allow it to be wet for about half a minute. It is better to wash your hair in the shower rather than the bath, as rinsing it in dirty, soapy bathwater will leave a film on the hair. A bit of warm water can be added to the shampoo so that it is less concentrated. Alternatively, you may want to dilute your shampoo by putting one part shampoo into an empty squeeze bottle and adding four to six parts water. It will clean just as well, last longer, and cost less; though don't expect as much lather, especially if your hair is oily. If you do dilute the shampoo and have oily hair, you may want to do two shampoos in a row. Avoid using too much shampoo. If you need more lather, it is better to add more water than shampoo. Remember that most lathering is created with synthetic detergents; more natural products that use yucca and soapwort as lathering agents may not lather as much.

Pour the shampoo from the bottle into the palm of your hand and work up a lather by rubbing your hands together before applying it to the oiliest portion of your scalp. Do not apply a big glob of concentrated shampoo to one place on your scalp, as it can be difficult to distribute. Touch your hands to several places on your scalp to distribute the shampoo evenly. Massage the shampoo into your scalp, starting from the roots of your hair and working toward the ends, beginning from the front of the hairline, above your eyebrows, toward the crown, using small circular movements. Then work from the side of your head toward the back, and last, through the arc at the nape of your neck. As the ends of your hair are the driest portions, they need less exposure to shampoo. Rather than dragging your fingers, use your finger pads to move your scalp in a gentle rotating fashion. Push your fingers together, then pull them apart while kneading your scalp; lift them when changing to a new area. If you have long hair, move your hands through the long portions at intervals. Handle your hair lovingly. It generally takes about two minutes to shampoo average-length hair, and three or more minutes if the hair is long.

Wash your hair in warm water and rinse it with cool water. Rinse well for longer than you think is necessary. Rinsing is imperative for removing all residues, which can attract dirt and cause scalp irritation. End with a final rinse of cool water to close the outer covering of the hair, making it flatter and better able to reflect light. Squeaky clean hair is a sign of damage and not something to strive for.

Scented Shampoo

Use any good-quality unscented shampoo.

4 ounces unscented shampoo
20 drops essential oil of your choice

Add the essential oil to the shampoo and shake until well combined.

Soapwort Shampoo

My daughter Sunflower and I run an herb camp for kids. This is one of the simple projects we made. We all had one of those hair days where everyone said, "Gee, your hair looks great!"

2 1/4 cups water
2 teaspoons soapwort root powder
2 teaspoons rosemary or chamomile flowers

Bring the water to a boil and remove it from the heat. Add the soapwort and rosemary. Cover and allow to steep 10 minutes. Strain into a bottle. Use for shampoo.

Yucca Root Shampoo

Yucca was used by ancient cultures in the southeast of North America as a soap. This doesn't lather like commercial shampoos, but it does leave the hair feeling thick and looking shiny.

2 cups rosemary or chamomile tea
2 tablespoons powdered dried yucca root

Combine the tea and yucca root, and use enough to work up a mild lather. Store the unused product in the refrigerator.

Dry Shampoo

There are some occasions when you may not be able to get your hair wet and you might need to know how to do a dry shampoo.

1 cup barley flour or arrowroot powder
1 tablespoon dried lavender, blended into a powder (optional)
2 drops essential oil of your choice

Thoroughly combine the ingredients. Work the mixture into the hair and scalp, as if you were washing the hair. Leave it in a few minutes so it can absorb oils. Bend over and brush out the powder (which will have absorbed the hair's oils and accumulated dirt), brushing one section at a time. You can do this outside or indoors with a towel placed underneath you.

Hair Conditioning

Conditioners have a positive charge and hair has a negative charge; this helps the conditioner to cling to the hair. Conditioners help retexturize hair and skin by providing a protective coating over the cells. This lubricates the hair shaft, promoting hair softness and helping to curb breakage and release tangles. Some conditioners coat the hair shaft, making the hair appear thicker. Most conditioners are applied after the hair is shampooed and rinsed. It is usually left on for two to five minutes, but it can also be applied before a shampoo in the form of a "hair mask" and left on for a minimum of twenty minutes to as long as overnight before being shampooed out. It is most important to apply conditioners evenly to the ends of our hair. Hair that is permed or colored will have more need for a conditioner.

There are many excellent natural hair conditioners on the market. Conditioners with a low pH are better for dry hair. Very thick conditioners can clog pores. If your hair is very fine, look for a liquid conditioner.

Even more intense than a conditioner is a pack, which is the answer for very damaged hair. They can be used twice a week. Common kitchen ingredients offer many possibilities for homemade conditioner hair packs. Here are some ingredients to consider (mash or purée them as needed): avocado, banana, beer, berries, carrots, celery, coconut water, coconut oil, honey, melon, olive oil, winter squash, and pumpkin. You can even use the pulp left over from making juice, and mix it with a bit of water. Someone once called me from a place where no conditioner was available. (Okay, it was a jail.) I suggested he use a bit of mayonnaise, which was available. Sea vegetables make excellent conditioner hair packs, as they stimulate hair growth, remove dirt and oil, and leave hair luxurious. First soak the sea vegetables for twenty minutes, then purée them in a blender.

You can make a scalp treatment oil with two ounces of jojoba oil or shea butter and one-quarter teaspoon of essential oil. Massage just a small amount of this mixture into your scalp. Wrap your head in a towel, and leave it on while you sit in the sauna or tub or lie on a slant board. Relax and take in the nurturing fragrance. Remember that most essential oils must be used diluted. Never apply them straight to your scalp, as this could cause irritation.

Apply the conditioner of your choice and wrap your head in a towel or cover your hair and scalp with a shower cap. Wait twenty to thirty minutes. Rinse thoroughly. If you feel your hair is overconditioned, it is probably due to insufficient rinsing.

Whether you buy or make your own conditioner, combing your hair with a wide-tooth comb, free of rough edges, while the conditioner is in your hair is very effective for dispersing the formula and preventing tangling. Afterward, cover your hair with a clean towel and leave the conditioner on your hair for ten to twenty minutes. If a sauna is available, that is a great way to spend this time; otherwise, just relax in the tub. Deep conditioning can be done overnight. When you are done conditioning, shampoo and rinse your hair to completely remove the conditioner. Light is reflected when the hair cuticle is closed, so ending with a cold water rinse can help make your hair more beautiful.

Scented Conditioner

Use any good-quality unscented conditioner.

4 ounces unscented conditioner
20 drops essential oil of your choice

Add the essential oil to the conditioner and shake until well combined.

If you (or more likely your kids) get chewing gum stuck in your hair, massage some peanut butter into the area and then shampoo it out.

Banana Conditioner

Your kitchen can provide ingredients for a nourishing and effective conditioner.

1 cup hot water
1 ripe banana
1/4 cup dried chamomile or rosemary
1 tablespoon coconut oil
1 tablespoon honey

Combine all the ingredients in a blender and apply to your hair. Leave on for at least 10 minutes, then rinse well.

Avocado Deep Conditioner

Avocados benefit dryness inside and out. This conditioner is excellent for dry and damaged hair.

1/2 mashed ripe avocado
1/2 teaspoon olive oil
3 drops rosemary or lavender essential oil

Combine the ingredients and massage into your hair and scalp, concentrating on the ends of your hair. Leave on for 10 minutes, then rinse well.

Hair Rinses

A rinse can be used after the conditioner has been rinsed out of your hair. Rinses make hair shinier and more manageable; they can also add highlights, restore the hair's acid mantle, soften the water, remove any soap residue, and promote a soft texture.

A simple rinse can be made with one-third cup apple cider vinegar for brunettes or one-third cup freshly squeezed lemon juice for blondes. Vinegar treats itchy scalp, dandruff, and dull hair and helps restore the scalp's natural acid

> Always rinse the hair well after swimming to remove salt and algaecides. The chlorine in pools is the same kind used to bleach clothes. It forms a bond within the hair's protein, eventually causing it to break down. Use a shampoo formulated to remove chlorine by converting it into a more water-soluble chloride, which is easier to rinse out. Natural food stores contain clarifying gels that are designed to remove chlorine and other chemicals from the hair.

mantle. You can infuse some of your fresh garden herbs into apple cider vinegar and create a super hair brew. Vinegar rinses are best for oily and normal hair rather than dry. White vinegar is ideal for blonde hair, apple cider vinegar for brunettes, and red wine vinegar for redheads. Be sure to use a vinegar that has at least 5 percent acidity.

Avoid using lemon juice on chemically processed hair, as it can be very drying. You can use herbs as a rinse by making a tea. Do not squeeze out the herb, or you will introduce too much sediment and make a cloudy product. Pour the strained tea slowly over your hair, including all of the scalp. Massage it in; don't rinse it out. Just let your hair dry, and enjoy the subtle radiance. Use homemade rinses within a day or two.

You can create a gentle final rinse for your hair by simply adding two tablespoons of vinegar or freshly squeezed lemon juice to three cups of warm water.

First, shampoo, condition, and blot hair dry with a towel; never rub, as this can cause breakage. Use dark-colored towels when using herbal hair rinses, or the towels may get discolored. You can lean over a sink or tub to apply the rinse. To be very efficient, the rinse can be collected in a basin and reapplied. Apply the rinse from a squeeze bottle, and distribute it evenly throughout your hair. Leave it on for at least five minutes if you are going to rinse it out. I prefer to leave it in. Any smell of lemon, beer, or vinegar will disappear upon drying.

Herbal Tea Rinse

Almost any herbs can be made into a tea to be used as a hair rinse.

1 quart water

4 heaping teaspoons fresh herbs of your choice

Bring the water to a boil. Add the herbs and remove from the heat. Stir, cover, and let rest for 1 hour. Strain into a large plastic squeeze bottle.

> Be sure to use clean jars and lids to store your homemade hair rinses. If you use metal lids, separate them from the jar with a layer of cut waxed paper; cut a circle a bit larger than the jar lid to prevent rust from developing when including vinegar in the product.

Herbal Vinegar

This can be used as a rinse to remove any soap residue and enhance highlights.

1 cup fresh herbs

2 cups vinegar

Place the herbs in a jar and cover with the vinegar. Place the sealed jar in the sun. Allow to steep for 2 to 3 weeks.

Herbal Hair Rinse

This combination of herbs and vinegar is the ultimate hair treat. It is excellent for dandruff, hair loss, and just plain beautiful hair! Use approximately one cup for each hair rinse.

- 1/2 cup nettle
- 1/2 cup rosemary (for brunettes) or chamomile (for blondes)
- 1 quart water
- 1 quart apple cider vinegar

Combine the herbs and water in a covered saucepan and simmer gently for about 10 minutes. Remove from the heat and steep at room temperature for 2 hours. Strain. Add the vinegar and transfer to a glass bottle. Store in the refrigerator.

Aromatherapy Hair Rinse

- 1 pint herbal tea rinse
- 2 tablespoons apple cider vinegar
- 4 drops essential oil of your choice

Combine all the ingredients in a glass jar or plastic squeeze bottle. Use immediately.

Basic Hair Rinse

This will make your hair radiantly shiny and remove any soap residue.

- 2 tablespoons apple cider vinegar or freshly squeezed lemon juice
- 3 cups warm water

Combine the ingredients in a glass jar or plastic squeeze bottle. Pour slowly through your hair and massage into your scalp for about 1 minute.

Herbal Aromatherapy Vinegar Rinse

The smell of vinegar dissipates as the hair dries, yet the lovely fragrance of the essential oil lingers on.

- 1 1/2 cups water
- 3 tablespoons fresh herbs
- 1/4 cup apple cider vinegar
- 5 drops essential oil of your choice

Bring the water almost to a boil. Turn off the heat and add the herbs. Cover, stir, and allow to steep for 30 minutes. Strain. Add the vinegar and essential oil.

Herbal Oil Scalp Treatment

This is fragrant and nourishing. During the time the treatment remains on your hair and scalp, you may want to give yourself a manicure, pedicure, facial steam, or mask. You can even leave the mixture on overnight, if desired.

2 tablespoons raw coconut oil or jojoba oil
15–30 drops essential oil of your choice

Soften the oil, if needed, by placing it in a cup and setting it in a pan of hot water (the water should reach just below the top of the cup). Stir in the essential oil. Pick up some of the oil mixture with your fingertips and massage your scalp. Repeat, covering the entire scalp, massaging in the oil for at least 3 minutes. Then work out to the ends of your hair. Cover your hair and scalp with a plastic shower cap and leave it on for a minimum of 20–30 minutes. Shampoo and condition.

Treatments for Sensitive or Irritated Scalp

- **Herbs for Irritated Scalp:** calendula, catnip, chamomile, or comfrey.
- **Herbs for Sensitive Scalp:** aloe, bay leaf, burdock root, calendula, chamomile, horsetail, marshmallow, nettle, or oregano.
- **Essential Oils for Sensitive Scalp:** cedarwood, clary sage, or ylang-ylang.

Aromatherapy for Healthy and Fragrant Hair

Employ the sensuous, attracting aspects of flowers, leaves, and roots to improve your mood and mental alertness and make your hair shine. The right essential oil can make you or those around you smile with delight whenever you brush your hair. You can put one or two drops of essential oil into the palm of your hand and rub it gently into the ends of your hair. Another way to use essential oils for hair care is to put one drop of oil into the amount of shampoo that you squeeze out for a single washing.

- **Herbs for Normal Hair:** chamomile, horsetail, rosemary, and sage.
- **Essential Oils for Normal Hair:** bergamot, Roman chamomile, geranium, lavender, orange, rose, rosemary, thyme, and ylang-ylang.
- **Herbs for Dull Hair:** basil, burdock, calendula, chamomile, cleavers, clove buds, cornflower, fennel seed, horsetail, linden flower, marshmallow root, mullein leaves, nettle, parsley, rosemary, sage, southernwood, and watercress.
- **Essential Oils for Dull Hair:** chamomile, juniper, lemon, and lemongrass.
- **Essential Oils for Fragrant, Mind-Blowing Hair:** jasmine, rose, rosemary, or ylang-ylang.

Dry Hair

Dry hair is often caused by a lack of sebum in the hair follicles and a lack of moisture in the hair shaft. Stress and menopause can be a contributing factor. Be sure to include some foods in your diet that contain essential fatty acids, such as freshly ground flaxseeds or raw flaxseed crackers. Protect your hair from the sun and avoid bathing in waters containing salt or chemicals. Avoid hair products that contain isopropyl or ethyl alcohol, which can further dry the hair. PABA helps shield hair from sun damage, thus preventing dry, brittle, or frizzy hair. It also helps blonde hair from oxidizing in a chlorinated swimming pool. Dry hair will benefit from the moisture of a humidifier, water fountain, or houseplants. When outdoors, protect your hair from harsh sunlight with a scarf or hat. Read about dry skin on pages 58–61 to learn more about promoting moisture from within.

- **Herbs for Dry Hair:** burdock root, calendula, chamomile, comfrey leaf and root, elder blossoms, geranium, horsetail, kelp fronds and other sea vegetables, lavender, lemon blossoms, marshmallow root, nettle, orange blossoms, parsley, patchouli, plantain, red clover, rosemary, sage, sandalwood, and southernwood.
- **Essential Oils for Dry Hair:** carrot seed, cedarwood, chamomile, clary sage, cypress, geranium, frankincense, geranium, jasmine, juniper, lavender, lemon, myrrh, palmarosa, peppermint, rose, rosemary, rosewood, sage, sandalwood, and thyme.

Oily Hair

Oily hair can be aggravated by stress and hormones, or it can be brought on by excessive conditioning. Brush your hair with a brush covered with a piece of thin muslin to absorb the oils. Eat a diet that is low in heated fats, such as dairy products, fried foods, chips, and bottled salad dressings. (Make your own fresh salad dressings with extra-virgin olive oil.) Use topical hair products that contain tea tree oil. (See the section on oily skin, page 61.)

- **Herbs for Oily Hair:** aloe vera gel, bay leaf, blackberry leaves, burdock root, calendula, chamomile flowers, clary sage, elder flowers, horsetail, kelp fronds, lavender flowers, lemon balm, lemongrass, lemon juice, linden flowers, nettle leaves, patchouli leaves, peppermint, raspberry leaves, red clover flowers, rosemary leaves, sage leaves, southernwood, green and black tea, thyme, witch hazel bark, and yarrow.
- **Essential Oils for Oily Hair:** basil, bergamot, cedarwood, clary sage, cypress, geranium, grapefruit, lavender, lemon, lemongrass, patchouli, peppermint, rosemary, sage, tea tree, and ylang-ylang.

Split Ends

This condition is called *scissura pilorum* and occurs when hair splits at the ends when individual cell layers separate from the older parts of the hair. The hair can split at any place along the hair shaft, not just at the ends. Hair with split ends is more prone to tangling. Chemicals and heat treatments can make hair more prone to breakage. The only solution is to trim the ends and avoid chemical treatments and damaging tools like hot rollers and blow-dryers. Shampoo less frequently, condition hair deeply, and eat a diet for hair health.

- **Herbs for Damaged Hair:** basil leaves, burdock root, calendula flowers, elder blossoms, frankincense, geranium, juniper berries, lavender flowers, mullein leaves and flowers, nettle leaves, parsley leaves, peppermint leaves, rosemary leaves, sandalwood, and southernwood leaves.
- **Essential Oils for Damaged Hair:** chamomile, geranium, lavender, peppermint, rosemary, and sandalwood.

Dandruff

Dandruff can occur from an excessively dry or oily scalp condition. Dandruff can also be the result of sensitivity to hair and scalp products (color, perms, sprays, conditioners, etc.) that may cause irritation, be the result of fungal overgrowth, or even occur from stress contributing to overproduction of the oil glands.

Simple dandruff (pityriasis) manifests as dry, flaky scalp, especially when the hair and scalp are brushed. The other type of dandruff is seborrheic dermatitis and results from overactive sebaceous glands that cause a more oily scalp; it can range from small, scaly dandruff to large patches. Stress, trauma, and illness will worsen cases of dandruff. The best remedies for dandruff are good nutrition and hygiene. Dandruff that is fungal related can be contagious, so avoid sharing towels, combs, hats, or other materials that come in contact with the head.

It is normal to experience some flaking of the scalp, but if it's excessive, perhaps your diet is too rich in sugar, fat, dairy products, and/or fried foods. A tablespoon of cold-pressed hempseed oil daily will help the body better metabolize fats and help balance both dry and oily scalp conditions.

In addition to the healthy-hair foods mentioned on page 97, broccoli and onions are both high in selenium, which helps curb dandruff from within.

Drink a quart of nettle tea daily. Zinc is often included in shampoos to relieve dandruff. Look for products that contain tea tree oil, which is antifungal. Selenium in dandruff products helps remove scalp buildup and control itching and flaking. As it can be slightly drying, be sure to get plenty of essential fatty acids in your diet. Sulfur, when used in dandruff products, can help restore damaged hair.

A folk remedy to treat dandruff is to combine fresh ginger juice with equal amounts of cold-pressed coconut oil. Apply the mixture to your scalp before bed and shampoo it out in the morning. Jamaicans rub aloe vera juice into the scalp until the dandruff disappears. In Burma, coconut oil is used in the same way.

- **Herbs for Dandruff:** artichoke leaves, burdock root, celery seed, clary sage, eucalyptus, horsetail, lavender, nettle, peppermint, quassia chips, rosemary, sage, southernwood, tea tree, thyme, and willow bark.
- **Essential Oils for Dandruff:** cedarwood, clary sage, cypress, eucalyptus, juniper, lavender, lemon, myrrh, patchouli, peppermint, pine, rosemary, sage, tea tree, and ylang-ylang.

Antidandruff Herbal Hair Rinse

Add apple cider vinegar if your hair is dry, or fresh lemon juice if your hair is oily. Use one cup of this rinse after each shampoo. Work it through your hair and scalp and don't rinse it out. Larger amounts can be made and chilled until needed, as results are best when this rinse is used over a period of time.

1 quart water
Large handful rosemary leaves
Large handful nettle leaves
Large handful thyme herb
Large handful lavender flowers
2 tablespoons apple cider vinegar or freshly squeezed lemon juice

Bring the water to a boil. Remove from the heat and add the herbs. Cover and let steep for 30 minutes. Strain and pour into a clean bottle. Add the vinegar or lemon juice. Store in the refrigerator.

Disappear Dandruff!

Try this along with making the healthful dietary changes suggested on page 97. Choose from the following essential oils: basil, birch, cedarwood, geranium, juniper, rosemary, sage, or tea tree. You can use a single essential oil or a combination of two or more. This can also be used as a deep conditioner that gets washed out thoroughly.

1/4 cup coconut oil
1/4 teaspoon tea tree essential oil or other essential oil of your choice

Combine the coconut oil and essential oil until well blended. Massage into your scalp before bed. Cover your pillowcase or wear a loose-fitting, breathable shower cap.

Antidandruff Aromatherapy Rinse

This works great!

1 cup water
2 tablespoons apple cider vinegar
5 drops rosemary essential oil

Combine the ingredients and apply to the scalp after every shampoo. Leave on for at least five minutes, but ideally just leave it in.

Hair Color

Hair color depends on the amount of melanin, a black pigment, which is made in the cortex of the hair shaft and sent to the hair root. Most melanin granules are elongated in shape. People with a large number of melanin cells tend to have dark hair, and those with a lesser number have fair hair. As we age, we produce less melanin, and our hair becomes lighter, even colorless, until it appears gray. Trauma, stress, nutrient deficiency, and genetic programming can all be factors in when and if hair grays. Hair that turns gray prematurely is said to be due to kidney deficiency and a lack of the enzyme tyrosinase. Graying usually begins around the temples and top of the head. Gray hairs are more likely to be coarse and wiry. Good foods for keeping your hair's youthful color include beets, black sesame seeds, blackstrap molasses, mulberries, nutritional yeast, and nuts. The Chinese herb ho shou wu means, in English, "Mr. Wu's hair stays black." In America it is sometimes called fo-ti. It is used by Asian cultures to help keep hair from turning gray. Copper, vitamin D, and the B-complex vitamins can help to keep gray at bay.

Hair Growth

Researchers now believe that the main storage center for hair renewal and growth is in a microscopic bulge alongside the hair follicle. My grandmother would say that if you want your hair to grow faster, cut it when the moon is waxing (getting fuller). Even if you want long hair, trimming it will help it look healthier by removing split ends.

Gray can be stunning. As we get older, lighter shades of hair create less contrast between our skin and hair. Dark shades look harsh and accentuate the imperfections in the skin.

Chemical hair dyes are alkaline and damaging to the hair. They cause the cuticle layer to expand so the color molecules can reach the cortex of the hair. Aniline dyes penetrate the cortex and last much longer than natural colors, but they also weaken the hair. Many hair dyes are toxic, and those that contain coal tar as a dye are suspected carcinogens. Exposing the hair to the chemicals used to bleach, dye, perm, and straighten the hair is going to compromise the health of your hair and can leave it more prone to breakage and split ends. A few years ago a hair dye marketed for men was found to contain lead, which can lead to nervous system disorders (including Alzheimer's). Pregnant women should be especially careful of exposing themselves to such chemicals, as should everyone else.

Natural food stores now carry ammonia-free colorings that color hair with herbs and other natural pigments. Natural hair colors are more acidic and coat the hair without penetrating it. Some folks even buy the natural products and bring them to their hairdressers, if they are not up for trying them at home. Better yet, find a salon that uses nontoxic products. Not only are these products safer for you and the environment, they also protect the health of the people who apply them and who are otherwise constantly exposed to chemicals in the conventional perms, colors, sprays, and straighteners that are commonly used. If you do decide to color your hair yourself, opt for lighter shades. Darker shades will leave your scalp showing through. A basic rule for a more natural look is to select a color that is one or two shades lighter or darker than your natural color. Anything more extreme should be done professionally. If you color your hair, consider your skin and eye color. Avoid selecting colors when you are looking at them under fluorescent lighting. Straying too far from what nature has given you will look artificial. But, then again, some of my best friends have happily enjoyed purple and pink hair.

If your hair turns green from chlorine, dissolve six aspirins into a pint of warm water. Massage it into the scalp and then shampoo it out. This is not a truly natural remedy, but swimming in a chlorinated pool is not natural either. A rinse with tomato juice will also help prevent the garish greenness. To get orange color out of the hair, such as from iron-rich water, add one-third cup of lime juice to your rinse water.

As we age, our skin gets one or two shades lighter. Therefore, if we choose to color our hair when we're older, a lighter shade will look more natural. Use the least toxic color available. Highlighting requires much less maintenance than dyeing and thus gives less exposure to chemicals. Since highlights have no defined root line, you can wait as long as six months before another treatment. Minimize jowls or a double chin by highlighting the hair around your temples and crown; this will draw attention away from the lower portion of your face. Highlighting the lower portion of your hair, especially if your hair is longer than chin length, can deflect lines around your eyes and/or mouth area. Experiment with some herbal rinses if you like to naturally highlight or darken your hair's color.

If you do color your hair, protect your scalp line with a coating of vegetable oil, and also be sure to protect your clothing. Avoid washing your hair the day after a color application; this will give the color a better chance to set in. Never color your hair when your scalp is broken or irritated. Trim your hair before coloring it, as there is no need to color hair that you are letting go of. It is best to only color hair that is already in good health. Avoid changing your hair color if you don't want to maintain it. You can, however, extend the time between touch-ups by avoiding hairstyles with a definite part. You can also find hair mascara sticks at beauty supply stores that can be used to touch up the roots.

Herbs and Essential Oils for Hair Color

- **Herbs and Other Ingredients for Dark Hair (these will darken hair and also maintain dark color):** apple cider vinegar, artichoke leaf tea (just use the leftover water after cooking artichokes), blue malva flowers, clove (use just a small amount or your head will feel numb), elderberries, henna, jaborandi, madder root, marjoram, mint leaves, nettle, plantain leaves, rosemary, sage, green or black tea, green or black walnut hulls, and yarrow tops.
- **Essential Oils for Dark Hair:** geranium, rosewood, and rosemary.
- **Essential Oils for Blonde Hair:** Roman chamomile, geranium, lemon, and eucalyptus.
- **Essential Oils for Gray Hair:** chamomile, lavender, rose, and sage.
- **Herbs for Blonde Hair:** calendula, chamomile, cornflower, green tea, lemon juice and peel, mullein flower, orange flower, red clover, rhubarb root, turmeric, and yarrow.
- **Herbs for Gray Hair (these will help darken the hair):** elderberry, nettle, rosemary, and sage.
- **Herbs and Other Ingredients for Red Hair:** alkanet root, beet powder, ginger, henna (avoid if getting a perm soon), hibiscus flowers, madder root, orange pekoe, paprika, red clover blossoms, Red Zinger tea, saffron, and sandalwood.
- **Herbs for White Hair (to enhance whiteness and brightness):** cornflower and chamomile.

Herbal Hair Lightener

This recipe has been used since the heyday of the Roman Empire.

3 fresh rhubarb stalks

2 cups water

1 tablespoon honey

Combine the ingredients in a blender, and process until smooth. Strain the mixture into a clean container. To use, massage the strained mixture into your hair (about 1/2 cup), cover with plastic wrap or a warm towel, and allow it to soak in for 30 minutes (the longer the mixture sits on your hair, the stronger the lightening properties). Rinse well.

Herbal Lemon Hair Lightener

This is lovely to try when spending time at the beach.

1 cup strong calendula or chamomile tea

1 tablespoon vodka

1 tablespoon freshly squeezed lemon juice

Combine all the ingredients, then strain into a spray bottle. Spray throughout your hair before spending time in the sun. Over time, it will have a lightening effect.

Highlight Lemon Rinse

This is the natural way to lighten hair.

2 cups water

1/2 cup freshly squeezed lemon juice

Combine the ingredients and work the mixture into clean hair that has been conditioned and blotted dry. Use before going out into the sun.

How to Henna Hair

Mix 1/2 cup of henna with 1/4 cup boiling water in a glass (not metal) container. Protect your hairline from getting stained by applying a coat of petroleum jelly. Apply the henna paste to clean, dry hair. Wear gloves when applying. Begin by brushing the henna onto your scalp at the back of your head. Continue parting your hair into sections, and applying the henna to each section, until your entire head is covered. Then, with a wide-tooth comb, work the henna through your hair, massaging it in. Cover your hairline with cotton. Wrap your hair in a plastic shower cap, and sit in a warm place for 15–45 minutes (the sun works great). The longer the henna sits, the more intense the color will be. Rinse well, then wash your hair using a mild shampoo. The color should last three to six months, depending on how often you wash your hair. It will gradually fade with regular washings without leaving a root line.

Hair Loss

When hair starts to fall out, it can be depressing. Sometimes the cause is genetic (androgenic alopecia). Hair loss can also occur from stress, sudden shock, physical injury, psoriasis, seborrhea, syphilis, a variety of drugs (such as anesthesia, blood pressure and cholesterol medications, beta-blockers, cortisone, X-rays and radiation, and ulcer medications), anemia, excessive dryness, fungus (ringworm), parasites, chemical and heavy metal exposure (copper is common), hormonal imbalances, systemic illness, diabetes, liver and kidney disease, thyroid deficiency, nutritional deficiencies (including anorexia and bulimia), and sudden or excessive weight loss. Chemotherapy chemicals impede the cell proliferation and division of hair. Tension can decrease circulation to the scalp and minimize nutrient availability.

Women often lose hair about three months after giving birth (but not during pregnancy) and after going off birth control pills. Excessive estrogen can contribute to hair loss. Hair loss from pregnancy and birth control pills usually reverses after about six months.

As far as genetic tendencies in men go, hair loss patterns typically follow the maternal rather than paternal side. In male pattern balding, the hair often recedes at the front of the scalp, the temples, and crown, on either side, or spreads out from the top. One frequent cause of male balding is excessive production of the hormones androgen and testosterone. Both of these hormones can cause the hair follicle to shrink. Even though genes play a part, you can slow or minimize the loss.

Sudden hair loss can be a sign of serious health changes and should be discussed with a competent health professional. To preserve hair, don't shampoo every day, as this will cause more hair to be lost.

Two of the leading types of hair loss in women are alopecia areata and the less common chronic telogen effluvium (CTE). Both are thought to be autoimmune conditions where the body's own system is attacking itself. CTE is suspected to be related to the hair follicles failing to move through their normal phases.

Alopecia capitis totalis is the loss of all scalp hair. *Alopecia universalis* is the loss of all body hair. Though *Alopecia universalis* is most common in men, it can also be experienced by women.

Natural medicine offers us much promise. Women and men may find that coloring their scalp with a soft eyebrow pencil in areas where hair is thin can minimize the visibility of hair loss until natural remedies have a chance to take effect. Here are some natural remedies you can try:

- Jojoba oil helps to dissolve imbedded sebum in the scalp. Look for jojoba-based hair care products.
- Spend about twenty minutes daily lying on a slant board to increase blood flow to your scalp. Alternatively, consider doing inverted hatha yoga postures, such as the shoulderstand or headstand. However, these are more advanced poses and should only be attempted by people who are experienced with basic hatha yoga. Find a class that suits your needs, with an instructor who can guide you.
- Wear your hair loose to avoid pulling at the scalp.
- Read the section on hair nutrition (page 97) and include these foods in your diet.
- Soybeans help to block the formation of dihydrotestosterone (DHT), a hormone associated with hair loss. They are best when fermented in the form of unpasteurized miso or Nama Shoyu (raw, unpasteurized soy sauce).
- Eat foods that tonify the kidneys, such as raw black sesame seeds, sea vegetables, and cooked black beans and kidney beans.
- Include silicon-rich foods, such as kelp and onions, in your diet. Eat the skin of organic cucumbers and red peppers for its high-silica content. Other good foods are oats, onions, nuts, buckwheat, barley, nutritional yeast, almonds, and seeds such as pumpkin and sunflower. Drink fresh vegetable juices made with beet, carrot, nettle, and spinach, with a bit of onion.
- Avoid heated fats and refined sugar.
- Hydrogenated oils are likely to clog the pores.
- Minimize your consumption of alcohol, caffeine, sugar, and refined carbohydrates.
- Supplements that may be helpful for hair loss are omega-3 fatty acids, beta-carotene, the B-complex vitamins, and zinc.

Herbs to Diminish Hair Loss

There are many herbs that have been used to improve hair growth and diminish hair loss. Mix a blend of the herbs of your choice and drink a quart of this tea daily.

- **Ashwagandha** nourishes the kidneys and adrenals, and thereby nourishes the hair.
- **Burdock root** is a nutritive herb that helps break up fatty deposits that can obstruct bodily functions, including those related to the scalp.
- **Dong quai** tea is especially good for women with hair loss.
- **Horsetail** is rich in the minerals silica and selenium, which help promote good scalp circulation.
- **Ho shou wu** is rich in minerals and is a kidney tonic and a rejuvenating agent.
- **Licorice root** prevents testosterone from becoming dihydrotestosterone (DHT), which is a substance believed to damage hair follicles. It may play a part in male pattern baldness by binding to the base of the hair follicles, causing them to shrink and deteriorate.
- **Nettle** is rich in minerals and tonifies the kidneys and blood.
- **Oat straw** and **oat seed** are mineral rich and provide nutrients the body needs for healthy hair, skin, bones, and teeth.
- **Rehmannia root** is a tonic that nourishes the kidneys, which govern hair.
- **Rosemary** improves circulation to the scalp and all other parts of the body.
- **Saw palmetto** prevents the conversion of testosterone into dihydrotestosterone, thus curbing hair loss in men.
- **Schizandra berries** were widely used among the royalty of ancient China as a youth preserver, beautifier, and sexual tonic. They nourish the kidneys, calm the liver, purify the blood, and promote radiant skin. They are both an astringent and demulcent, having the ability to both dry and moisten the system as needed.

Super Hair Smoothie

You can drink this smoothie daily to help promote hair growth!

1 cup raw almond milk

1 ripe banana

1/2 cup raw pumpkin seeds

1/2 teaspoon sea kelp

1 tablespoon nutritional yeast flakes

1 tablespoon raw agave syrup

Combine all the ingredients in a blender and process until smooth. Drink immediately.

Folk Remedies for Hair Loss

- If the hair roots are still alive, rub a clove of garlic or piece of onion (preferably when sleeping alone) over your scalp before bed to increase circulation and encourage hair growth. (Do not leave the garlic clove in contact for long with your skin, as it can cause blistering.) The scalp can be warmed first with a steaming towel for this remedy to be even more effective. Shampoo and condition in the morning.
- Dip peeled fresh ginger in brandy and rub it over the balding area.
- Mix castor oil with equal amounts of fresh onion juice. Cover the affected area with the mixture and leave it on overnight. Do this every night for two consecutive weeks.
- Apply tincture of cayenne to the balding area of the scalp. Keep it away from your eyes and mouth.
- Apply aloe vera gel to the scalp till it tingles fully. This is believed to stimulate the hair follicles and promote thick, full hair.
- I personally know three men who have told me the following remedy worked for them. Buff your fingernails against each other in a circular motion. Do this for five minutes at a time, three times daily. This sure beats biting your nails and is also said to help slow down hair loss and graying.
- Other folk remedies to use to stimulate hair growth and stop hair loss include applying fresh stinging nettles to the balding area of the scalp by lightly beating them onto the head. Be aware that this can cause a rash and irritation that lasts up to twenty-four hours, yet it can be very helpful. I will go so far as to say that gently whacking the scalp with fresh stinging nettle plants will stimulate scalp circulation better than any product on the market and can be virtually free, should you have a nettle patch out back. I would normally never suggest such a harebrained idea, except it is a valid part of European herbal practice, and my own beautiful husband has done this many times since 1978 and still has the most radiantly beautiful hair.
- Let go of negative thought patterns. Rather than saying, "I'm losing all my hair," try "I'm taking better care of myself. My hair will grow thick."
- Bald can be beautiful, and many people choose this as a hairstyle. Celebrate the many forms of beauty.

Trichotillomania is a mental condition where those afflicted feel compelled to pull out their own hair. Look into hypnosis and herbs to help calm anxiety, such as St. John's wort, lemon balm, and oat straw. Replace a negative habit with a positive one. For example, instead of picking at your hair, give yourself a scalp massage or learn to do a craft with your hands.

Hair Loss Tonic

This is to be applied to the scalp and left on.

1 cup water
1 cup aloe vera juice
15 drops clary sage essential oil
10 drops rosemary essential oil

Combine all the ingredients and store in a tightly sealed glass jar.

Nettle Hair Tonic

Apply the mixture nightly to the scalp before bedtime to prevent hair loss. After massaging, brush the hair well. Or use as a final rinse without washing it out.

1 quart vodka or apple cider vinegar
2 cups fresh nettle, washed and chopped
1/2 cup rosemary
1/2 cup sage leaf

Combine all the ingredients in a large glass jar. Cover and allow to stand for 2 weeks, shaking the mixture daily. Strain. Store unused portions in the refrigerator for up to 1 week.

Herbs and Essential Oils to Help Hair Loss

- **Herbs and Other Ingredients for Hair Loss:** aloe, basil, burdock, eclipta, honey, nettle, parsley, rosemary, sage, and yarrow.
- **Essential Oils for Hair Loss:** basil, cajeput, carrot seed, cedarwood, clary sage, cypress, eucalyptus, juniper, lavender, orange, peppermint, rosemary, sage, thyme, and ylang-ylang.

Hair Removal

Hair occurs everywhere in the skin except the palms of the hands and soles of the feet. I am all in favor of the natural look, but hairy underarms and legs are not everyone's cup of tea. I compromise and shave only in the warm months and go *au naturel* during the cooler months when I'm wearing more clothes. To avoid any redness if you choose to shave, use a good topical lotion and apply a fragrance-free moisturizer afterward. I like cold-pressed raw coconut oil.

Sugaring

One natural method of depilation is a process using sugar. Mix one tablespoon of sugar with an equal amount of water. Melt over gentle heat in a pan over the stove. Allow to cool; when it reaches body temperature, apply it to your skin using a spatula, pressing it into your skin with a piece of cotton fabric. Allow it to set, and then pull it off by lifting the cotton, pulling against the direction the hair grows. Rinse with cold water. The area sugared should be smooth for about eight weeks. Sugar is easier to clean up after than wax.

Styling

Your hairstyle should be balanced with the rest of your body, following your hair's natural growth patterns. When cut, hair makes an excellent compost addition: fertHAIRlizer.

Bending over while you comb or brush hair will increase body. You can apply a light-hold spray before coming back to a standing position for longer-lasting volume.

Rather than perming your hair, cut it and style it to give more volume. Layered hair creates a fuller shape that enhances facial features. Shorter hair exposes more of the facial features. Long hair really can be worn by people of any age, provided the hair is healthy. Bangs can accentuate the eyes; however, if bangs are too long, they will accentuate the nose instead.

Pipe cleaners can be used to give hair a natural wavy look. While your hair is damp, take strands and twist them around the pipe cleaners.

Avoid wearing your hair in a tight, constrictive style or sleeping in tight rollers, which can impair circulation, cause headaches, and weaken hair. Severe, pulled-back styles can also draw more attention to facial imperfections. If a ponytail is what you need to keep hair out of your way, consider doing a low, side ponytail. With this style, the hair is out of your way but still softening to your appearance. If you do pull your hair back, a bit more makeup can be flattering, and having a bit of hair framing the face can make women appear younger. For special occasions, feel free to delight in hair art and ornaments. It's fun to braid hair when it is slightly damp. The next morning you will have mermaid waves. I also like to put fun accessories into my hair, such as barrettes (I love sparkly ones), scarves, fabric hair ties, tiny braids, hair magnets, or whatever is your style or fashion statement. I recently bought some glow-in-the-dark sparkles in Haight-Ashbury. Can't wait to try them out!

When I noticed that my teenaged daughters were spending outrageous amounts on hair care products, we tried making a few of our own.

Aloe vera gel can be used as a styling gel. Its high zinc content is beneficial for hair. It also can tighten the scalp and curb excessive oil production. Two to three tablespoons of honey can be dissolved in warm water and used as a styling gel. Flaxseed tea can also be used as a setting lotion or styling solution. The natural sugars and protein it contains help thicken the hair. Another effective styling gel can be made by putting flat beer into a spray bottle. Once it dries, the beer smell will disappear.

For hair-spray buildup (which is less likely with natural brands), add one tablespoon of baking soda to the amount of shampoo you put in the palm of your hand (don't use more than this, as it can be drying). Use this only when needed. Spraying hair before styling gives it a softer appearance; styling then spraying can result in a stiffer look. Avoid hairstyles that require electric rollers or curling irons for daily maintenance. Subjecting the hair to these treatments too often will certainly result in damage to the hair.

My friends Ellie, Vujika, and Eagle have done a truly beautiful thing with their hair. They grew their hair, cut it, and then donated it to Locks of Love, a nonprofit organization where hair is made into hairpieces for financially disadvantaged children who have lost their hair due to medical conditions and treatments.

Locks of Love
2925 10th Avenue North, Suite 102
Lake Worth, Florida 33461
www.locksoflove.com

Lemon Hair Spray

When my daughters brought home a $20 bottle of hair spray from the health food store, I decided to show them both how to make a hair spray at home.

Juice of 1 lemon (3–4 tablespoons)
1 cup distilled water
1 tablespoon vodka (as a preservative)

Combine all the ingredients and pour into a pump bottle. Refrigerate between uses. Keeps for about 1 month.

Flaxseed Styling Gel

This is the other hair spray we learned to make. It's been used for thousands of years!

1 tablespoon flaxseeds
1 cup water
1 tablespoon rose or orange flower water
1/2 teaspoon vegetable glycerin

Soak the flaxseeds in the water for 15 minutes. Strain the seeds out and discard them (if you throw them in the yard, you may be rewarded with lovely blue-flowered flax plants). Add the remaining ingredients to the liquid and pour into a spray bottle. Apply a small amount when styling your hair. Store the unused portion in the refrigerator.

BEAUTIFUL HANDS AND NAILS

Our hands are an extension of our heart, brain, and respiratory system, according to Asian medicine. Hands are one of our most expressive features. They serve us as tools and provide the joy of sensory touch. Busy hands help us eat, work, grasp objects, and play; they can easily become rough and dry. Despite their importance, they are often ignored. Our hands are almost constantly exposed to the elements, being subject to heat, cold, wind, water, and a barrage of chemicals. Hands and nails can be a good indicator of health. Hands are one of the first places on the body to show age. The skin on the backs of our hands is some of the thinnest and is likely to show our age faster than any other part of the body except our face. Both men and woman appreciate not being touched by rough skin.

Everyday Care of the Hands

- Hold your hands in elegant postures. Practice *mudras* (mudras are symbolic hand gestures used in religious ceremonies and dances of India and in yoga).
- In Asia, a graceful position for hands at rest is for them to be held unobtrusively, the fingers close together, curling slightly inward, with one hand resting atop the other, like sleeping birds or seashells.
- Avoid carrying heavy packages, which can enlarge the veins of the hands. Use handles on bags rather than keeping parcels held in tightly clenched hands. Don't carry more than you need to. Put parcels down to rest, and at intervals, hold your hands over your head to balance circulation.
- During the colder seasons, wear gloves or mittens to prevent chapping.
- Protect your hands from chemicals by wearing waterproof gloves when doing housecleaning.
- Use natural biodegradable products for household chores.
- Before gardening, scratch your nails into a bar of soap; this will help keep the dirt out. Wearing gloves when gardening will also help protect your hands.
- Avoid using your nails as tools. Use your fingers, not your nails, to pick up objects.
- If you are doing lots of office work, use tools, such as letter openers.
- Type with the pads of your fingers rather than the tips.
- Wash your hands in warm water rather than hot, which can damage growing cells.

- Be sure to dry your hands thoroughly, including between the fingers where fungi can grow and chapping can occur. (Asian medicine says that keeping hands wet too frequently can be a factor in arthritis.)
- Keep a bottle of natural lotion next to the sink as a reminder to use it after washing and drying your hands. Have some lotion in your desk, purse, and briefcase, and use it as needed throughout the day. Massage lotion into your hands before bed.
- Massage your hands and also exercise them. Share hand massages with loved ones.
- Hot hand baths can be used to relieve writer's cramp, arthritis pain, and improve circulation. Add two to four drops of rosemary or sage essential oil to a basin of warm water to relieve soreness. Chamomile hand baths are good for eczema.
- You can exfoliate your hands by massaging them with sugar and a bit of almond oil or some powdered rolled oats. Rinse well. A gentle hand scrub can be done with 1 teaspoon coconut oil and 1 tablespoon raw sugar. Massage well into your hands. Rinse well with cold water.

Daily Exercises for Your Hands

- Shake your hands vigorously to increase circulation and bring nutrients to your nails.
- Do a wrist stretch by extending one arm in front of you. Point your fingers toward the floor while using the other hand to gently pull the hand toward you. Feel the stretch in your wrist and forearm. Now do the reverse, pointing the fingers upward. Do both steps on the other side.
- Consider buying a set of Chinese hand balls, which are available at many natural food stores.
- Press your hands together as if praying, only harder. Relax. Repeat ten times.
- Separate and stretch your fingers ten times.
- Take a rubber band and alternately place it around your thumb and each individual finger as you stretch wide.
- If your nails are slow to grow, take up knitting or typing.
- Practice The Rose exercise. This is done by clenching your fist tightly, like a young rosebud. Then gradually open it, as if the rose were blooming. Stretch, stretch, stretch. Then totally relax.

Nail Diagnosis

Observe your fingernails. In Asian medicine, the "Liver" governs the nails. The fingernails also correspond to peripheral circulation in the upper body. Use your left hand for doing nail diagnosis. The newer growth will be at the nail base. Nails should be slightly dome shaped; if they are very flat, the lungs may be weak.

Thick nails indicate calcification and/or excess protein. When the nails are thin, you may need more minerals and B vitamins; you may also have difficulty assimilating protein. Brittle nails indicate lack of nutrition and poor circulation. Nails that peel and chip indicate either a lack of protein or poor assimilation of it.

Nail color reflects the quality of the blood. Pink nails are the healthiest color. Pale white nails are an indication of anemia. Try pressing the nail; if the color doesn't return immediately, anemia is even more likely. White spots on the nails often indicate a zinc deficiency, excessive consumption of sugar, or that the nail was injured. If the flecks are on the right hand, the problem is more physical; flecks on the left hand correspond more to emotional problems. Red-colored nails may mean high blood pressure. Bluish-tinted nails may mean the heart and lungs are not functioning optimally and that perhaps metals, like copper or silver, are in the body in excess. Low blood pressure and lack of oxygen may also be a factor. Nail fungi can indicate a selenium deficiency.

continued

Rich Hand Cream

Do something lovely for your hands that do so much for you!

1 cup raw coconut oil
50 drops essential oil of your choice

Combine the ingredients with a fork. Store in a clean, dry glass container.

Growing Strong Nails

Nails are made of keratin, like hair. Keratin is a strong fibrous protein that is produced by cells beneath the cuticle at the nail's base. Like the epidermis of the skin and hair, nails are made primarily of protein cells. As the nail grows out from the matrix, and as new cells build up and die, the nail is pushed forward and out the surface. Nails grow about 1/250 of an inch daily, or about half an inch every four months. (This is one-third to one-half as fast as hair.) Nails grow quicker in summer than winter and more so between the ages of eighteen and twenty-eight; they also grow fast during pregnancy and when the body is in a state of healing. The nails on your dominant hand tend to grow faster than on the hand you use less often. An adult nail can take eight to nine months to grow, whereas a child's nail can take three to four months. Fingernails grow about twice as fast as toenails. In Asian medicine, the health of the nails depends on the health of the "Liver" system. It is the nails' matrix, under the skin, that is very much alive. The white crescent of the nail is called the lanula, and it is part of this matrix.

The best nail hardeners are nourishing food: fresh fruits and vegetables and raw nuts and seeds. To nourish the nails from the inside, eat more oats and include sea vegetables in your diet. Drink three cups of horsetail tea daily, which is rich in the mineral silica. If your nails are very brittle, include three tablespoons of freshly ground flaxseeds to your regimen. Essential fatty acids can improve hand and nail quality.

The word "manicure" is derived from the Latin word *mani*, meaning "hand." Share a manicure with a friend. Clean nail implements and change files often. Don't allow a manicurist to treat you with equipment that hasn't been sterilized.

All nail polishes are nothing more than refined versions of automobile paint. Nail polish can dry and stain the nails as well as limit oxygen exposure to the nails. If you do use one for special occasions, look for those that are free of toluene and formaldehyde. Brands such as No Miss, Sante, and Firoze are free of the most toxic ingredients and available at natural food stores. Remove any moisturizer that may be on your nails or the nail polish will not adhere to them. Polish in layers, allowing each layer to dry between coats. Three coats are considered standard. Don't dry nails with a blow-dryer or other heat source or the polish will lift from the nails. Always treat the nails diligently after polishing. Polishing your nails with a buff gives them a natural shine and keeps them beautiful without artificial polish.

All nail polish removers are hazardous to the health of nails, and of all the cosmetics available, they are one of the most allergenic. Acetone, an ingredient in most nail polish removers, is more harmful than acetate. Artificial nails can harbor high levels of bacteria. Using nail polish remover can contribute to ridges in the nails, and it can be especially damaging to the entire nail and cuticle. Wipe off any old nail polish with a cotton ball saturated in acetone-free nail polish remover. Use as little as possible. Hold it on the nail for about fifteen seconds. Never soak your nails in it. The fumes are toxic, so be sure to put the lid back on the bottle right away and work in a well-ventilated area. Start at the base and work upward to the tip to avoid pushing polish and remover into the delicate cuticle.

To make your nails stronger, soak them in warm olive, sesame, or wheat germ oil with four drops of lemon essential oil for ten minutes. Or soak your nails in mashed kiwifruit, green papaya, or pineapple for ten minutes; your nails will benefit from the natural enzymes found in these fruits. Soaking hands in buttermilk helps to fade brown spots. (To learn more about treating brown spots on the backs of your hands, see page 70.) If your hands are stained, add a bit of fresh lemon or lime juice and use a gentle brush. Soaking nails in horsetail and nettle tea will strengthen both the nails and cuticles.

Spoon-shaped nails (concave) can be a sign of a need for more chromium and other minerals. Vertical nail ridges indicate exhaustion of the nervous system and liver. Some hand readers say that deep vertical lines can indicate chaotic eating habits, environmental changes, and possible intestinal parasites. Fever can cause wide nail depressions. Birth control pills can cause nail brittleness. Some people have ruts on their nails. If the ruts are at the nail base, adrenal weakness may be a factor. Ruts in the middle of the nail indicate pancreas weakness. Ruts at the top indicate thyroid weakness. In general, nail grooves indicate poor digestion.

Swelling around the cuticle area indicates excessive consumption of sugar, fruit, juice, drugs, and perhaps a systemic yeast overgrowth. People who bite around their cuticles may have repressed sexual energy or are going through a crisis. Hangnails can be a sign of extreme eating patterns, anger, frustration, passion, and intense emotions.

Nail Biting and Other Bad Habits

Biting nails and cuticles can cause swelling and redness and make us prone to infection of the hands. Nail biting can also cause dental problems. Biting the nails can be an indication of stress and/or a calcium deficiency. Use calcium supplementation. Applying tea tree oil or aloe vera gel on the fingers has been used as a bitter deterrent for nail biters.

Any activity that alters a person's mood has the potential for abuse: television, telephones, video games, computers, shopping, driving too fast, exercising, overspending, religious fanaticism, gambling, playing the lottery, stealing, and going to meetings are just a few examples. People can even become addicted to habits, such as playing with their hair, biting their nails, and picking at their skin. Humans are notorious for habits such as hair pulling, scratching, blinking, pencil chewing, and teeth grinding. These habits are often unpleasant, unhygienic, and irritate those around us. Most addicts of this sort are trying to escape from boredom in their lives. These types of behavior stimulate endorphin production in a way that is similar to many drugs. These habits become addicting when we rely on them to calm ourselves. All mood-altering activities tend to initially produce a sense of euphoria.

Make a list of the reasons why you should stop your bad habits. Put it where you can read it often—above a sink, on a mirror, as a bookmark, in your wallet. Being clear about why you want to give up a habit is very important.

continued

Occasionally soak your hands in warm herbal tea, such as calendula, chamomile, or fennel, or simply add about five drops of essential oil to a basin of warm water; this will help relieve soreness and relax the hands that do so much for us. Beware of commercial nail-strengthening products. Many contain drying ingredients, including formaldehyde and toluene. After soaking, with your nails still oily, buff them in one direction with a piece of natural fiber cloth. Spend about one minute on each nail.

Not everyone agrees on whether nails should be cut while wet or dry. Water softens nails, and cutting soft, water-logged nails can make them more susceptible to tears and damage, but they are less brittle. Use manicure scissors or nail clippers. When your hands are totally dry, file your nails with an emery board. To create beveled nails, file from underneath in one direction from each side toward the center. Use a paper emery board to gently round your nails, rather than making them sharp and pointed. It is best to keep all of the nails at the same length. Sawing back and forth weakens the nails and encourages splitting. After clipping, file gently with an emery board with a "down and away" stroke, filing in one direction from front to back. Filing the corners weakens the nails, so avoid that. Pointed talons haven't been in style in most countries for a long time. The shape to strive for is a squared oval, as this best protects the nail's growth. The nails can then be buffed in one direction, avoiding the cuticles, to increase circulation.

The nail's cuticle is the protective layer of skin between the matrix and the outside environment. I don't understand why people feel they need to manipulate the cuticle by pushing it back or cutting it. This only creates potential nail problems, such as weak, rigid, brittle, peeled, dented, or unevenly growing nails. Never cut the cuticle, which protects the nails by sealing off the opening between the skin and nail. Instead, gently massage the cuticles whenever you apply hand lotion; this will keep them pliable and less likely to crack.

You can't expect a book called *Beauty by Nature* to endorse artificial nails. Fake nails can cause horizontal grooves to develop close to the nail's cuticle. The nail plate can also thin when the acrylic nails are removed and cause our own nails to separate from the nail bed, a condition we could all live without called onycholysis. Artificial nails can harbor high levels of bacteria and wearers are more prone to nail infections.

Natural Nail Treatments

- Wash your hands in soapy water. Scrub your nails with a soft nailbrush to increase circulation. A small nailbrush is a good way to keep them looking clean. Then immerse your hands in clean water that contains two drops of chamomile essential oil.
- Buffing your nails against each other is a great way to build nail strength.
- To prevent nail fungus, minimize sugar, fruit juices, and alcohol in your diet. Use zinc as a supplement. Apply tea tree essential oil to the area.
- To help with nail discoloration, moisten a cotton swab with vinegar and apply to your nails for one minute.

Nail and Hand Salve

Rub this on your nails, cuticles, and hands. This formula will keep for three to four months without refrigeration.

4 tablespoons olive oil
2 tablespoons grated beeswax
2 tablespoons cocoa butter
1 tablespoon shea butter
20 drops geranium or rosemary essential oil

In a double boiler or a small saucepan, warm the oil, beeswax, cocoa butter, and shea butter just until the wax has melted. Remove from the heat, pour into a container, and allow it to cool a bit, but do not cover. When slightly cooled, add the essential oil and stir. Put the lid on when it is completely cool.

Develop a strategy for stopping. If you do catch yourself indulging in the habit, say Stop! aloud to yourself and later under your breath. Every time you catch yourself engaging in a bad habit, write it down in your day-timer. Wear a loose elastic band around your wrist and snap it hard every time you indulge.

Have someone photograph you indulging in your addiction or habit while you look into the camera. When you get the photo back, look at it carefully and ask yourself what it is trying to tell you. Put all that extra energy into doing something good that helps society and yourself.

Whatever part of your body is involved in the habit (nails, hair, skin, etc.), do something different and more positive with it. For example, instead of biting your nails, buff them, or instead of picking at your face, massage it. Play with toys for a few minutes, such as Play-Doh or Chinese hand balls. Keep these tools where you are likely to need them.

Be consistent and keep track of your progress. Consider showing your progress chart to someone you really trust. Let them know you are not asking them to nag you, and tell them in what ways they can best help you. Reward yourself. For example, if you go all day without engaging in a habit, put one dollar or five in a piggy bank so that you can buy something special.

Decide to change. Refuse to be enslaved by anything. Learn to deal with any lapses in a positive, healing way. Be a free, conscious being. Habits are automatic; the way out of them is to remember the way out.

Nail Oil

Nourish your nails with this simple formula. It's great for toenails, too!

2 tablespoons castor oil
1 tablespoon olive oil
2 drops lavender essential oil
2 drops cypress essential oil

Combine all the ingredients, bottle, and label. Shake and apply to your nails before bed.

Cuticle Cream

Use this to massage into the cuticles to keep them soft.

2 tablespoons coconut oil
$^1/_2$ teaspoon cocoa butter

Combine the ingredients in a small saucepan, and warm over very low heat, stirring constantly. Store in a clean container with a lid.

BEAUTIFUL FEET

If you walk barefoot upon the morning dew, you will become beautiful.

—AMERICAN FOLKLORE

Our feet support us, ground us, and connect us to the earth. On an emotional level, they represent our foundation, security, and inner strength. Our feet bear the weight of our entire bodies approximately 1,500 times for every mile we walk. (Another good reason to lose extra weight.) Each foot contains over 7,000 nerve endings, 107 ligaments, 19 muscles, and 26 bones (a quarter of all the bones in the body). According to Dr. Scholl's, the average person walks about 115,000 miles in a lifetime. That's far enough to circle the planet almost five times! For many people, feet are a low priority when it comes to the care and attention we give our bodies. Many think that just having some shower water drip onto our feet is all that's needed. And yet, all it takes is an irritation on the tiniest toe to give discomfort to our total being. Here are a few ideas to let our feet know we appreciate them.

- Stand with your weight balanced on both feet rather than all the weight being placed on one side. Feel connected and supported by the earth. Drop your shoulders.

• Many foot problems are due to poor-fitting shoes, including narrow toes and high heels. No wonder women are more prone to foot problems! Make sure your shoes fit well and don't cause unnecessary pressure. Avoid buying shoes in the morning, as the feet expand during the day, and what fits perfectly at 10:00 a.m. may seem too tight by 6:00 p.m. When trying on shoes, wiggle your toes to make sure there is sufficient room. Try on both shoes, as most people have one foot that is slightly larger than the other. A proper pair of shoes should fit well from the get-go; don't expect them to stretch out. Your foot size may change or widen as you get older. Good-quality shoes, not the ones with the cheapest price tag, are essential! High heels can cause posture problems, as they create a forward lunge and shorten the hamstrings. If you walk to work, or to the subway or bus, wear sneakers and then change into other shoes for work, if needed. Should you don a pair of high heels for a special occasion, do it for no more than three hours, and slip them off now and then. (I love to dance barefoot!) Don't force your children to always wear shoes. Bare feet allows foot muscles to grow stronger and builds coordination. Wear natural-fiber socks and change them often. Choose shoes made of natural materials that allow your feet to "breathe." Alternate the shoes that you wear so your shoes have the opportunity to air and dry out between each wearing. Avoid synthetic shoes without ample ventilation; otherwise, the shoes will trap moisture and promote fungus and odor. The least problematic shoes tend to be flat, open, quality slip-on clogs. Pour some dried beans into a shoe and walk for a few minutes as a foot-massage exercise. Remove your socks and shoes after exercising. Air your feet out in the sun for short periods of time. Go barefoot when it is safe and practical.

Footbaths

After being on our feet all day, it feels delightful to soak them in a basin of warm water to which essential oils or herbs have been added. Beneficial essential oils for the feet include bergamot, camphor, German chamomile, clary sage, eucalyptus, geranium, lavender, lemon, orange, peppermint, rose, rosemary, sage, spearmint, and tea tree. Footbaths can be very therapeutic for odoriferous or aching feet; they can also help reduce cellulite, swelling, calluses, leg cramps, and varicose veins. A footbath before bed can aid sleep. Footbaths can be alternated between hot and cold. Massaging your feet while soaking in hot water is delicious. Footbaths are great to administer before a foot massage. Cold footbaths can relieve upper-body congestion, as the blood rushes down to heat the lower part of the body.

For a footbath, use 1 teaspoon fresh or dried herbs per gallon of water, or 5–15 drops essential oil to 2 gallons very warm water. The recipient of the footbath should be dressed, though uncovered below the knees. A cool washcloth can be placed on the forehead and refreshed every two to three minutes. At the end, pour cold water over the feet (top and bottom). Dry the skin thoroughly, and put on clean socks. Herbs that can be used in footbaths include the following:

- **Catnip herb** relaxes stressed feet.
- **Chamomile flowers** help relieve sore, swollen feet.
- **Eucalyptus leaves** are invigorating and deodorizing.
- **Gingerroot** warms feet that feel chronically cold. (Ginger footbaths are also good for gout and headaches.)
- **Horseradish** is good to use during a cold or flu, as it is decongesting.
- **Horsetail herb** reduces perspiration.
- **Juniper berry** is antifungal.
- **Lavender flowers** refresh tired feet.
- **Lemon peel** invigorates tired feet.
- **Lovage root** is a strong natural deodorant.
- **Marjoram herb** invigorates tired, achy feet.
- **Marshmallow root** softens rough feet.
- **Mustard seed** warms feet that feel chronically cold. Use mustard when you have a cold, flu, or congestion.
- **Peppermint herb** is stimulating for tired feet and cooling to hot feet.
- **Pine needles** are refreshing and deodorizing.
- **Rosemary herb** is deodorizing and relieves soreness.
- **Sage leaves** are antiperspirant and deodorizing.
- **Thyme leaves** are antifungal and refresh tired feet.

To use the herbs in a footbath, simply prepare a tea. Bring one gallon of water to a boil, remove from the heat, and add sixteen heaping teaspoons of the herb. Cover and allow to steep for ten to twenty minutes. Strain. Soak your feet in a basin of the warm tea. A simpler alternative is to add five drops of essential oil made from any of the above plants.

Other kitchen remedies to add to a footbath include one-quarter cup of any of the following:

- **Apple cider vinegar** is antifungal and deodorizing.
- **Baking soda** is deodorizing and detoxifying.
- **Bran** cools burning feet.
- **Epsom salts** relax tired, achy feet.
- **Salt** footbaths are detoxifying.

Some people find it helpful to fill a container with marbles and walk around in it to take the ache out of their feet. Plunge your feet into a cold bath filled with just an inch or two of water and five drops of peppermint essential oil when the goal is to revive and refresh yourself.

Foot Massage

A foot massage feels heavenly! You can give one to yourself or show the one you love just how pleasurable this can be, then you can trade. Natural food stores carry helpful foot massage tools. I especially like foot rollers and keep one by my desk to roll on my feet while I write.

A simple exercise for weak feet and tender ankles is to put twelve marbles on the floor. Pick them up one by one with your toes, and drop each one into a cup. Try towel curls. Place a small, open towel on the floor. With your toes, grasp one end of the towel, curling it under your foot. Continue gathering it till the opposite end is reached. Repeat five times on each foot. Flex your ankles back and forth, and practice clockwise and counterclockwise rotations several times daily. Spend some time with your feet elevated by lying on a slant board, or spend a few minutes a day in the shoulderstand or headstand yoga posture, if you are adept.

Athlete's Foot

You don't have to be an athlete to suffer the itching irritation of athlete's foot. Those who frequent public pools, gyms, and shower rooms; get exposed to prolonged moisture; sweat a lot; wear tight, nonbreathable shoes; or are prone to nail injuries and cuticle damage are the most likely to develop this problem. Be aware that this fungal infection can easily be spread, so avoid sharing pedicure tools like nail clippers. This disorder is actually a form of ringworm, which thank goodness is not a worm at all but a species of fungus, *Trichophyton mentagrophytes*. It is seven times more prevalent in men than women and is more common where conditions are hot and humid. Since most authorities believe that it is easily spread, wear rubber thongs when showering in public places. Athlete's foot can be a symptom of yeast overgrowth in the body. Sugar, fruit juice, alcohol, and yeasted breads may all contribute to a yeast overgrowth. Take a probiotic supplement. Try soaking your feet in three quarts of warm water to which one cup of apple cider vinegar has been added. You can also massage a handful of coarse salt into your feet. Dry the feet well, especially between each toe, and apply some tea tree or lavender essential oil to the affected area; both are excellent antifungal agents.

Antifungal Foot Soak

Don't despair! Try this instead.

1/4 cup apple cider vinegar
5 drops tea tree essential oil
5 drops lavender essential oil
1 gallon hot water

Combine the vinegar and essential oils. Add to the water. Soak your feet for 10 minutes. Dry thoroughly.

Antifungal Foot Powder

You can apply this morning and night to fight fungus.

1/4 cup bentonite clay
10 drops tea tree essential oil
10 drops geranium essential oil
10 drops lavender essential oil

Combine the ingredients and store in a glass jar. Liberally apply to affected areas.

Being overweight can lead to many foot concerns, such as fallen arches, bunions, odor, and misalignment of the bones. Too much weight contributes to the wear and tear of the feet. Improperly fitted shoes can cause blisters. Soak the affected area in a bucket of hot water to which one-half cup Epsom salts have been added. Then apply an antiseptic cream. Apply straight lavender oil to the blister.

Bunions are localized swelling or bony bumps (inflammation of the bursa), often on the sides of the toes, especially the big toe. They are sometimes hereditary. Tight shoes can cause this otherwise painless ailment to become irritated. Cushion the area with a foam pad when wearing shoes. An anti-bunion exercise is to loop a big rubber band around the big toe, then pull the toe away from the smaller toes, holding each pull five seconds. Repeat ten times. Practice spreading your toes, which can easily be done in the bathtub. Poultices that can be applied to bunions include grated lemon peel or chopped onion soaked in apple cider vinegar and held in place overnight by a bandage. Castor oil can also be applied to bunions.

A callus refers to hardened skin, similar to a corn, often on the ball or heel of the foot. Calluses are caused by the way we walk or by pressure on the foot from shoes at odd angles. Walking barefoot in the sand or grass helps to soften the feet and is a great exercise. (Avoid this practice if you have diabetes.) You may want to insert insoles into your shoes to cushion the area. Use a foot scrub of one-half cup sea salt and one-half cup baking soda. Garlic oil can also be applied to calluses. Apply fresh lemon juice to a corn or callus.

A corn is when the skin over the toe forms a hard protective coating, usually due to pressure. Corns and bunions can be softened by soaking the feet in warm salt water for ten minutes and then using a pumice stone (made of lightweight volcanic ash) before applying castor oil twice a day to the afflicted area. For corns, an alternative folk remedy is to tape the inside of a fresh lemon peel to the area overnight for several nights in a row. Be sure to choose shoes that fit well and don't cause unnecessary pressure. Try Epsom salt foot soaks for bunions, calluses, and/or corns.

Ingrown toenails usually occur on the big toe and can impair walking. Avoid wearing shoes that crunch your toes. Soak the affected foot in hot water, and then apply a healing herbal salve. Do your best to keep the skin away from the nail by using some athletic tape to gently pull and secure the skin away from the toe. To prevent this ailment, be sure to cut your toenails straight across rather than in a sloping fashion.

Some foot problems may be due to sports injuries or overexertion. Arnica oil can be applied to sprains and bruises. It is best to not apply it to broken skin as it may be irritating. Take arnica homeopathic pellets internally for strains, swellings, and ligament and soft tissue injuries. The homeopathic remedy *Rhus toxicodendron* can be used for torn ligaments and injuries to the joints and tendons. Consider homeopathic *Hypericum perforatum* for toe injuries. Use *Ruta graveolens* for heel tendon injuries, sprains, and bone bruises.

Metatarsalgia is an irritation of the heads of the metatarsal bones. When people who are afflicted press on the balls of their feet, pain is felt. The pain may be due to pressure, pinched nerves, flat feet, arthritis, or stress fractures. The metatarsal bones support about 60 percent of our weight. Wearing well-cushioned shoes can help.

Foot odor can often be improved by taking three capsules of chlorophyll daily; chlorophyll is a natural deodorizer. Put fresh sage leaves in your shoes for sweeter-smelling feet.

Heel pain is known as plantar fasciitis; it is often felt when we take our first steps in the morning. The name refers to the ligament band that runs from the ball of the foot to the heel. Try rolling your foot on a golf ball. Another beneficial exercise is to stand on the bottom stair while facing upward. Hang either one or both heels over the step edge while supporting your weight with the handrail and feeling the stretch. Hold for thirty seconds. Repeat several times.

Plantar warts (*Verruca plantaris*) appear on the soles of the feet and are spread by an easily transmissible virus. They are characterized by a distinct black or brown pinpoint that will hurt or bleed if squeezed. (A corn will not.) Soak plantar warts in hot salt water. Many people report that applying castor oil or tea tree or orange essential oil twice a day to planter warts can help them to disappear. Also effective is to tape the inside of a banana peel to the area, which can even be done under socks and shoes. Vitamin E by itself or a paste of vitamin C and water can be applied to a plantar wart. Warts can be filed down. It can be interesting to check out the reflexology chart on the facing page to see what corresponding organ the wart is related to.

If your feet are cold and you feel that their circulation is poor, adding warming spices such as cayenne, cinnamon, or ginger to your diet may help. Constantly cold feet may be a sign of insufficient circulation, fibromyalgia, or hypothyroidism. Tingling and numb toes may be a symptom of a B-vitamin deficiency.

How to Give Yourself a Pedicure

The word "pedicure" means "caring for the feet." Remove any old polish (should there be any) with an acetone-free nail polish remover. Soak your feet in warm water or in an herbal tea or kitchen remedy soak (see page 128) for fifteen to twenty minutes. Scrub with a nailbrush to clean out dirt lodged under the nails. Use a wet pumice stone or exfoliating scrub, such as cornmeal, ground almonds, salt, or sugar. (Using a pumice on corns may cause further irritation.) It is best to do this in a bath or shower, after the skin has been somewhat softened by the hot water. Don't expect all of the dead skin to go away with one session; it works best when repeated regularly. The skin on the soles of the feet is ten times thicker than any other portion of the body. Dead skin cells tend to build up more quickly on the heels and balls of the feet.

Dry your feet thoroughly. Trim your toenails straight across after soaking, as they will be softer and easier to cut. Buff the nails in one direction, avoiding the cuticles, to encourage a healthy glow by stimulating circulation. Polish if you like with an acetone-free polish. Let it dry thoroughly. Massage a rich lotion into the feet. For cracked feet, massage coconut oil into your feet and put cotton socks on before bed.

Foot Scrub

Delight yourself or your beloved with this treat. This can also be used on rough elbows and knees.

3 tablespoons sea salt

2 tablespoons extra-virgin olive oil

10 drops essential oil of your choice

Combine all the ingredients. Apply in small rotating circles to dampened skin.

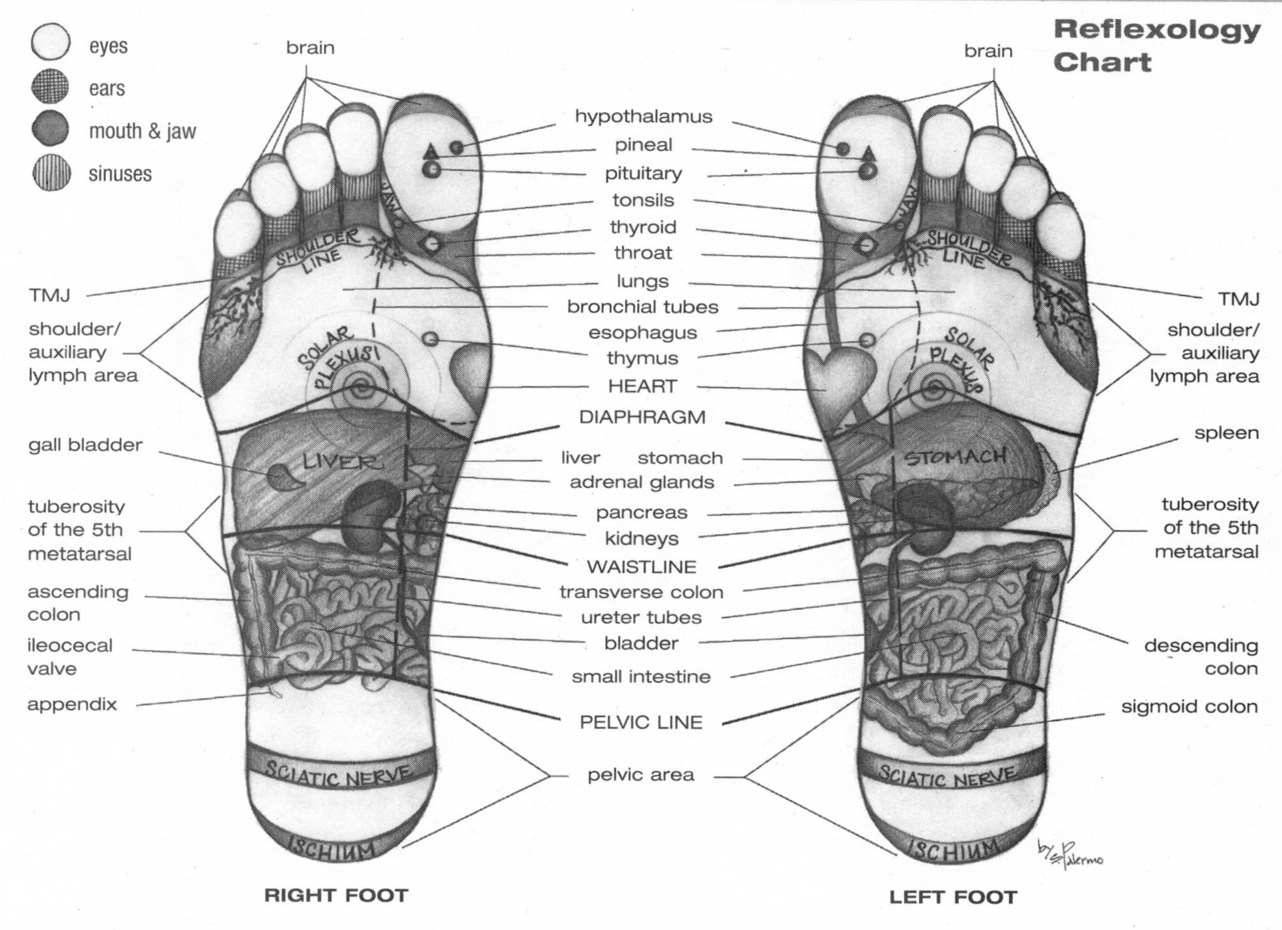

To order this poster in full color, contact gracebodywork@yahoo.com.

Foot Powder

Avoid commercial products that contain talc. They can be harmful to your lungs.

- 1/4 cup baking soda
- 10 drops sage essential oil
- 10 drops tea tree essential oil
- 10 drops peppermint essential oil

Combine all the ingredients in a glass bowl using a fork. Store in a clean, dry glass jar.

Antifungal Drops

This might be just what you need to treat athlete's foot or other foot problems.

2 teaspoons tea tree essential oil
2 teaspoons lavender essential oil
2 teaspoons eucalyptus essential oil

Combine all the ingredients in a one-ounce dropper bottle. Place a drop or two on fungal-infested areas morning and night (or more often, if desired). Rub it in well.

BEAUTIFUL AND HEALTHY BREASTS

Breasts are unique and beautiful. They play a role in love and nurturing. It gives us much joy to share our breasts in pleasure and connection with lovers and babies. Tactile tissue is, after all, what furthers the continuation of life! The right breast is said to be linked to external events and issues related to masculinity. The left breast is associated more with inner events and issues with femininity. Repressing anger and creativity can create tumors in the body. For breast health, it is important to express feelings and "get things off your chest."

Breast health is related to the health of the entire being. Pay attention to the health of your liver and keep your colon functioning well. Improve lymphatic circulation with exercise. Low thyroid function can impair the liver's ability to break down extra estrogens.

Breasts can still grow past puberty until the early twenties. In our twenties, breasts are composed of fat, milk glands, and collagen. Pregnancy can cause nipples to become darker; this enables color-blind babies to spot them more easily.

Much of breast shape is due to genetics. It is normal for one breast to be larger than the other (often the left). Fluctuating hormonal levels can cause breasts to change shape and size. Midcycle, estrogen levels are highest and can increase breast sensitivity. The week before the moon time, progesterone and estrogen levels are high and breasts may be more tender, hard, bumpy, or swollen. As we age, our glands can shrink and collagen is replaced by fat. Sleeping on your stomach can cause breasts to become misshapen over time.

Eat five servings of fruits and vegetables daily. Include plenty of dark leafy greens and sea vegetables in your diet, as they help drain and disperse congestion. Learn to make flax crackers out of whole fresh raw flaxseeds. Raw pumpkin seeds are an excellent breast enhancement food. Avoid meat, eggs, and milk products, especially those tainted with synthetic hormones. Get off of heated oils for breast health (fried foods, baked goods, and chips are not the ideal food for breast health and beauty). Herbs that have long been used internally as breast enhancement teas and pills are usually made from fennel seeds, fenugreek seeds, and saw palmetto berries. Rosemary is an excellent antioxidant herb to use in moderation. In ancient Egypt, women ate nigella seeds to firm and beautify their breasts. A few minutes a day of sunshine and air is also great for breast health.

Breasts are thin-skinned compared to the rest of the body. Breast massage is a way to love and nurture yourself as well as to improve circulation and lymphatic drainage. If you use a cream or lotion on your breasts, make sure it is free of preservatives and made with fresh unheated oils. Coconut oil scented with a few drops of essential oil can be used to massage the breasts. The massage oil can be scented with essential oils of cypress, geranium, juniper, lavender, rose geranium, and/or rosemary. You can add seven to ten drops of any of these essential oils to your bath, and be sure to turn over to soak your breasts in the tub when bathing. End baths and showers with cold water, or at least a splash over the breasts. French women insist this helps inspire a perkier bosom. A folk remedy to keep the breasts firm is to apply lady's mantle compresses to the breasts. Essential oils (dilute them first with a carrier oil) that are massaged into the breasts to increase their size include clary sage, geranium, or ylang-ylang, all of which contain phytohormones.

Sagging Breasts

After nursing two babies, I was sure my children had consumed the lovely shape of my teenaged figure. After doing The Deer exercise below for about six months, my husband and I noticed that my breasts had been restored significantly. Several friends and even my own mother asked if I had gotten implants.

Regular exercise of the pectoral muscles, which support the breasts, can help stop droopiness and create the appearance of cleavage. Rowing, basketball, weight training, and Nautilus machines all support breast health. Some people might prefer push-ups and chest presses. Engage in moderate exercise at least twice a week.

Basic Pectoral Exercise

Lie on the floor with weights in each hand. Bring the weights together above your chest and hold for two seconds. Repeat seven times.

The Deer Exercise

One of the most important exercises from the Taoist tradition for long life and sexual vitality is called The Deer, also known as stoking the Golden Stove. The Deer moves blockages of energy, helps honor the vulnerable parts of our bodies (the breasts and testicles), stimulates hormonal production, and relieves a

Kegel Exercise

Both men and women should do Kegel exercises, also known for thousands of years by those knowledgeable about Tantra as root locks, or *mool bandha*. Kegels build libido, strengthen muscles weakened by childbirth, and increase pelvic muscle support. Exercising these muscles releases tension and improves circulation in the pelvic area. Kegel exercises massage the prostate gland and improve vaginitis, cystitis, infertility, and incontinence. They give the vagina a tighter grip. Kegels can also help men differentiate between orgasm and ejaculation. Within just a few weeks, Kegels can improve women's orgasms and help men have greater staying power. And they are free!

Kegel exercises are done by tightening and then relaxing the muscles that control the flow of urine. If you can't figure out how to do this, practice during urination by starting and stopping the flow of urine. Inhale while contracting, exhale while releasing. Start with twenty-one contractions and work up to one hundred contractions three times daily. Practice daily, alone, or with your beloved. These are very private exercises that can be done while reading, waiting for the traffic light to change, or even while riding in a crowded elevator. You can do Kegels when making love, to delightfully squeeze your beloved with your love muscles.

wide range of reproductive disorders. This exercise can also help prevent prostate problems, hemorrhoids, and erectile dysfunction. There is a male and female version.

For women, sit up straight and place the heel of one foot gently against the clitoris. Rub your hands together to warm them, and massage your breasts (not the nipples) in a slow, circular motion thirty-six times. If you want the breasts to grow larger, make inward circular movements. If your breasts are overly large, tender, or prone to lumps, massage them in a counterclockwise direction thirty-six times. If you want to maintain the same breast size and tone your breasts and promote their health, do one direction in the morning and the other direction before bed. Then lower your hands and do thirty-six deep Kegel exercises (see sidebar). Women can take a break from The Deer during their menses.

For men, The Deer is performed sitting or standing. Rub your hands together to warm them. Hold the scrotum with one hand, and with the other palm massage right below the navel in a circular motion eighty-one times. Then switch hands and directions and massage again. Follow with thirty-six Kegel exercises.

The Deer is done morning and night. It is essential to focus on the exercise and not think about what you're going to wear or have for lunch. Be present.

Bras

No other part of the female anatomy is as constricted as the breasts and the lymphatic tissue in that region. Though bras might not cause cancer, they may be a trigger for it. Women who sleep with bras are more likely to get breast cancer than those that don't.

Stop the madness! Use either cotton or other natural fibers to protect this vulnerable part of our bodies. Spandex, a common fabric used in bras, can contain chemicals like phenolic acid, known to cause skin problems. Avoid bras that change your natural shape with breast-shaping components and underwires. Strapless bras are especially tight around the armpits, compared to other bras. Go braless, if that suits you. At least reduce the amount of time each day a bra is worn.

If you have nipple hairs, it is normal. If they are unwanted, you can either wax the area or tweeze them out after cleansing the area with an antibacterial agent, such as witch hazel; wipe the area again afterward.

To occasionally create cleavage when wearing a special outfit (or attending the Grammys), tear off a piece of half-inch-wide adhesive tape, long enough to cup both breasts from one underarm area to the other. Use one arm to cradle your breasts and push them together as you tape. Use a bit of blusher in the cleavage area, if you like.

Look for any changes in your breasts. Get attention for nipples that suddenly become inverted, red, inflamed, swollen, or have a discharge, including bleeding.

EYE HEALTH AND BEAUTY

If eyes were made for seeing, then beauty is its own excuse for being.

—Ralph Waldo Emerson

It is said that the eyes are the windows to the soul. No facial feature adds to our beauty and sparkling vitality more than the eyes. The precious gift of sight, which brings light and color into our lives, is worth all the attention we can focus toward achieving and maintaining healthy vision. All organs give the purest part of their energy to the eyes, helping to create their alertness and brightness.

To keep our eyes strong or improve them, it is important to express our emotions and not allow pressure to build (causing glaucoma) or cloudiness (causing cataracts). Crying can actually be a therapeutic way to clean and heal the eyes.

In Asian medicine, the "Liver" system governs the eyes, and many ocular disorders have their roots in liver disharmonies. The liver meridian passes through the eyes. For example, insufficient blood supply to the liver or liver heat can be the cause of eyes that feel dry. Eyes that are often irritated and bloodshot may be due to the liver being irritated by coffee, alcohol, and chemicals. For bloodshot eyes, dab cotton balls in rose water, place over closed eyes, and lie down (slant boards are great for this) for fifteen minutes.

The kidneys govern the function of vision, and eye problems are also associated with deterioration of the kidneys. Acute eye conditions, such as a watery discharge, are likely to be associated with the lungs and allergies. Eyes that have a discharge of mucus may be aggravated by a diet too rich in congesting fats.

The eye area tends to be more prone to allergies and also tends to show wrinkles before other parts of the face.

Spend at least twenty minutes daily in full-spectrum light, preferably in the early morning before rays are too harsh, without glasses or contact lenses, as light enters the eyes and affects the pituitary and pineal glands. During the day, spend time looking at the healing green colors of nature. Consider using full-spectrum lighting in your home and workplace. Natural light improves visual acuity and helps prevent eyestrain.

Glasses can help us see clearly, but they don't actually improve vision. If you wear contact lenses, do so conscientiously by cleaning them properly and removing them to let your eyes breathe as much as possible. If you always wear glasses or contact lenses, consider that you may be blocking nature's full-spectrum lighting as well as available oxygen to the eyes. When it is safe and can be done without strain, try to spend a little time each day without anything covering your eyes. Close your eyes and allow the sunlight to rest upon your closed eyelids for three to five minutes.

Another beneficial eye-strengthening technique is called "sunning." It is done by standing or sitting with closed eyes (though no glasses or contacts). Turn your head gently from the left to the right, allowing the early morning or evening sun's rays to gently cross over your closed eyes. This is best done outside, preferably when surrounded by the calm, cooling green colors of nature.

Cheap sunglasses filter only some rays but allow other rays that may be harmful to come through. The best sunglasses are gray, green, or brown, in that order. Do limit sun exposure.

Simple walking twenty to forty minutes daily is also good for the eyes. Protect your eyes from excessive heat and toxic chemicals; even those that are inhaled can affect the eyes. Several times a day, splash cold water over your eyes to improve circulation. An ancient folk remedy to benefit the eyes is to gaze at the cooling rays of the moon. Sleep in a well-ventilated room. Sleep on your back, as sleeping all crunched causes creases leading to permanent lines. Using two pillows to elevate your head will keep fluids from pooling around your eyes.

When reading or focusing your eyes for long periods, squeeze your eyes shut for a few seconds to increase blood flow to the area. If you spend your days looking at close objects, take a break every half hour or so and gaze off into the distance. Why not have a mandala, a collage that you make every year that inspires your goals, hopes, and dreams, a beautiful window view, or other inspirational things to gaze upon.

If you spend your days in front of a computer, keep the room lighting low and the screen three to four times brighter than the room. Minimize glare by keeping the computer monitor away from light sources, such as windows. Consider using an antiglare screen. Make sure characters on the screen stand out sharply. Have the screen positioned fourteen to twenty inches away from your eyes, just below eye level. The colors of display characters that are easiest on eyes are amber and green. Fifteen minutes out of every hour try to do some work away from the computer.

You might also try wearing a patch over one eye and spending some time roaming your yard or drawing for short periods of time to exercise one eye at a time.

Acupressure on the feet, with special attention to the bottom of the second and third toes, can benefit the eyes. If your eyes need some extra help, you may want to massage the correlating reflex points at the base of the bottoms of the second and third toes in a firm circular motion. Deep massage at the base of the neck may help to relieve tension that impairs vision by moving energy in the liver meridians.

Foods that are particularly beneficial to the eyes include raw sunflower and black sesame seeds, beets, carrots, celery, green leafy vegetables (especially kale, spinach, and watercress), leeks, sweet potatoes, barley, blueberries, dates, lycii berries, mulberries, raspberries, and raisins.

Spirulina, a beneficial superfood rich in beta-carotene and DHA, can be added to smoothies. Use chervil, cilantro, paprika, and parsley frequently as condiments. Garnish your meals with fresh organic marigold or calendula petals from your garden, which are rich in lutein, a nutrient that promotes eye health.

Bright Eye Smoothie

Nourish your eyes with this antioxidant-rich drink. Other good juices to mix into this smoothie are beet, celery, endive, parsley, or spinach.

1 cup fresh carrot juice

1 cup water

1/4 cup unsalted raw sunflower seeds

1 tablespoon spirulina powder

Combine all the ingredients in a blender and process until smooth.

Herbal eyewashes have been used for centuries to strengthen the eyes and improve vision. Eyewashes can be used for tired, inflamed, or infected eyes. Splash your eyes with cold water. Hold the top half of your head in a bowl of cold water so that your eyes are in the water but your nostrils are not. Open your eyes under the water. Eyecups can also be used. This causes the blood vessels of the eyes to contract and then relax. This is excellent to practice when your eyes are getting lots of use from reading or sitting in front of a computer. Only use herbs that are traditionally used for eyewashes, such as chamomile flower, cornflower, elder flower, eyebright herb, fennel seed, raspberry leaf, red clover blossoms, or rue herb. The amount of herb needed for an eyewash is a little less than is used for tea. Some people claim that eyewashes can even improve vision.

Always use a fresh eyewash to avoid introducing bacteria into the eyes. Whatever is not used in one treatment should be refrigerated and then allowed

Tips for Selecting the Most Flattering Eyeglasses

- When trying on glasses, wear any eye makeup you usually do so you can see the effect. Look for lenses large enough to allow eye makeup to be visible.
- Select frames that rest above your eyebrow. If your brows show over the glasses, you can look surprised.
- Avoid large, dark-colored frames if you are pale or don't want to wear makeup, as the glasses will be too overpowering.
- If you have lots of wrinkles and need a strong eyeglass prescription, select a small frame or the eyeglasses will magnify every line.
- If your features appear downward, select glasses that have their upper portion slanting up and outward.
- Square frames can draw attention away from sagging jowls.
- If you have puffy undereyes, select rounder, thicker frames rather than thinner ones. Thin wire-type frames will not conceal puffy undereyes.
- If you have a long nose, select frames that sit low on your nose.
- If your face is round, select oval frames that are longer than they are wide. If they angle at the corners, it will be even more flattering.
- If your face is long, choose round angled frames that are wider than they are long.
- If your face has a sad appearance, frames so large they droop onto the face will make you look sadder.
- Wearing lipstick when you wear glasses will help make your face look more balanced.

to reach room temperature, or warmed slightly, before using. Especially in cases of eye infections, it is important to sterilize the eyecup between use either by running it through the dishwasher with a heated dry cycle or by filling the cup with boiling water for one minute and then discarding the water.

Place one scant teaspoon of herb in a cup of distilled water and simmer at a low boil for ten minutes to ensure sterility. Cool the herb tea to body temperature before administering. Be sure to use a very fine strainer (a coffee filter is excellent) to avoid getting particles of the herb in your eyes. Pour the well-strained tea into a sterilized eyecup. Lean back and pour the mixture into the eyes, being sure to blink several times so the eye is well bathed. Then lean forward into a sink to catch the excess solution, and repeat with the other eye.

Nutritional therapy for poor eyesight is a good place to begin, but it is also necessary to distribute these valuable elements throughout the body with proper exercises. Eyes should get exercise just like any other part of the body. Eye exercises can increase circulation and tonify the six muscles attached to our eyeballs.

An Exercise to Improve Vision

Doing this exercise daily has greatly improved vision for many people, including myself.

1. Keeping your head still, look up and down 7 times. Close your eyes to rest 10 seconds.
2. Look from one side to the other 7 times. Close and rest 10 seconds.
3. Look diagonally from one direction to the other 7 times. Close and rest 10 seconds.
4. Look diagonally from the opposite direction to the other 7 times. Close and rest 10 seconds.
5. Roll your eyes in an upper half circle and back 7 times. Close and rest 10 seconds.
6. Roll your eyes in a lower half circle and back 7 times. Close and rest 10 seconds.
7. Place the backs of both hands over your closed eyes and rest for one full minute.

Another simple way to exercise your eyes is to hold a finger or pen ten to twelve inches away from your face, focus on the tip, then look off into the distance. Repeat several times. Turn your head from side to side as if saying "no" emphatically.

Puffy Eyes

Puffy eyes can be an indication of a food allergy, sinus problems, weak kidneys, sulfites in wine, alcohol consumption, excess sugar consumption, crying, or exhaustion. If the puffiness disappears as the day wears on, fluid retention may be the cause, which is related to the kidneys. Drink nettle tea on a regular basis, but avoid drinking it before bed. Avoid allergens, which can even be part of your bedding, such as a down pillow or comforter. Adequate rest is paramount. Be sure to remove all makeup before bed and make sure what you are using is not causing an allergic reaction. Sleep on fluffy pillows. A folk remedy to reduce eye puffiness is to make a small pillow (about eleven by fourteen inches) filled with dried chrysanthemum flowers. Place it inside another pillowcase and put it inside your pillow at night. Make a fresh pillow every season, if it helps you.

Be sure you aren't using an eye cream you are allergic to. Eye creams are designed to be richer and thicker than other moisturizers, as the area around the eyes lacks oil glands. Avoid putting any creams or moisturizers too close to your eyes, as they can cause puffiness.

Try sleeping with an extra pillow to elevate your head and keep less fluid from pooling in the undereye area.

An exercise for puffy eyes is to squeeze both eyes shut tight. Draw the lids inward toward your nose without using your hands. Keep your eyes relaxed. Then move your eyelids outward. Hold for three seconds. Repeat seven times. This exercise works quickly. Start doing it every night for ten nights. Then reduce the frequency to three times a week.

Home remedies for puffy eyes include lying down (on a slant board if possible) with a slice of raw peeled potato (red ones are best), apple, cucumber, or melon over each eye. Also helpful is to apply cool, moistened tea bags over the eyes. Chamomile, cornflower, elder flower, eyebright, marshmallow root, peppermint, and/or black tea can be used.

When your eyes feel tired, irritated, and swollen, rather than resorting to synthetic eyedrops, which give only temporarily relief and can lead to more irritation later, consider some gentler approaches. Beware of heavily chlorinated pools or swimming in unclean waters, which can cause eye infections or irritations. Wear watertight goggles, if necessary.

Dark Circles and Red Eyes

Dark circles under the eyes can be due to allergies, sun damage, natural pigmentation, or even shadows that are cast, making this area appear darker. Would you believe that a quart of nettle tea daily also benefits this condition?

Red irritated eyes can be due to lack of sleep, exposure to smoke, alcohol consumption, allergies, makeup particles, dryness, air pollution, staring at a computer all day without a break, or overuse of eyedrops. Use a humidifier, blink regularly, and avoid wearing contact lenses all the time.

Keep the undereye and crow's-feet areas moist, as there are no oil glands in this part of the face. The skin of the eyelids is some of the thinnest on the body. Smile when applying eye cream to observe just how far the crow's-feet extend. Apply a lightweight eye oil or cream to the upper lid also. Avoid applying masks to the eye area, as the skin is too fragile to be subjected to any mask that causes tightening. Eye creams are not really that different from moisturizers for other parts of the face.

May your eyes enjoy the wonders of the world and be a reflection of your inner health and beauty!

If your eyes are begging for attention, it makes sense to take a few moments to give them some genuine nurturing. There are some Swiss homeopathic eyedrops on the market that work very well. Remember that when our eyes are giving us trouble, we should look to the cause of the problem and do our best to remedy it. For a proper diagnosis, please consult with a competent, preferably holistic-oriented ophthalmologist for problems such as seeing colored rings around lights; blurred or double vision; seeing imaginary spots, lines, or flashes of light; or burning, watery, or itchy eyes.

BEAUTIFUL TEETH AND BREATH

Be true to your teeth or they'll be false to you!

—OLD FOLK SAYING

Tooth Powder

This is an excellent toothpaste that improves many dental and gum conditions.

1/4 cup baking soda
20 drops peppermint essential oil
20 drops tea tree essential oil

Combine all the ingredients and store in a clean glass jar with a lid. To use, sprinkle a small amount on a damp toothbrush.

Tooth Whitener

This can be used once a month.

1 teaspoon baking soda
Food-grade hydrogen peroxide

Add just enough of the hydrogen peroxide to the baking soda to make a paste. Use to brush your teeth for 2 minutes. Rinse well.

Gum-Strengthener Blend

Treat your gums with a combination of massage and essential oils.

3 tablespoons vodka or apple cider vinegar
8 drops myrrh essential oil
8 drops tea tree essential oil
2 drops peppermint essential oil

Place all the ingredients in a small glass jar and shake well. Massage a few drops into your gums to promote healthy teeth and gums.

Receding Gums Blend

You can entice gum tissue to regenerate.

1/2 cup chopped yerba mansa
1/2 cup chopped echinacea root
1/4 cup myrrh tears
1 cup chopped prickly ash bark
Vodka or apple cider vinegar, as needed

Place the herbs in a glass jar and cover to the top with either vodka or apple cider vinegar. Add an extra inch of the liquid so the herbs are totally submerged. Shake daily for 1 month. Strain (I like to use a clean piece of muslin), pressing the herbs out. Compost the herbs and bottle the remaining liquid. Massage into the gums after brushing.

Flavored Toothpicks

Use good-quality undyed wooden toothpicks. Place the toothpicks in a small glass jar, big enough for the toothpicks to fit into. Cover with essential oil (suggested oils include anise, cinnamon, fennel, ginger, peppermint, orange, spearmint, or tea tree), and allow the toothpicks to absorb the oil overnight. Remove the picks with tweezers and place them on a plate to air-dry. Store them in an airtight container. Use the toothpicks to clean your teeth, stimulate your gums, and freshen your breath. Some people I know say these have helped them to quit smoking! Any leftover essential oil can be reused for another project.

Beautiful Breath

The prettiest face and figure can be spoiled by offensive breath. It is difficult to smell our own breath, as our noses adapt to whatever smells they are constantly exposed to. If you are in doubt about your breath quality, ask someone close to you to rate your breath. I have a deal with my best friend. We are supposed to tell each other if either of us has bad breath. Now that we are both raw foodists, however, bad breath rarely happens.

Find out what the cause of bad breath is and correct it. It could be due to eating a food you are allergic to (like dairy products), constipation, detoxifying the body, some medications, tooth or gum problems, poor lung health, or eating onions or garlic. When the mouth is dry, such as in the morning from not having had any water in several hours, saliva production decreases and can contribute to bad breath.

In the morning, get up to brush your teeth before kissing your partner. Brush your tongue as well as your teeth. Bacteria can collect on the tongue, so brushing your tongue or using a tongue scraper is also a good idea and will get rid of twice as much bacteria as simply brushing your teeth. You can use a specially designed tongue scraper or simply a soupspoon for good oral hygiene. Just insert the spoon upside down and press the edges into your tongue. Rub it across the surface several times, then follow with a rinse of cool water. Use a refreshing mouthwash. See the next page for ideas for herbal mouthwashes.

Keep a glass of water by your bed to quench nighttime thirst. If you still suffer from bad breath, drink green vegetable juice daily made with wheatgrass or parsley. You can also take three chlorophyll capsules daily. Apples and celery are natural breath fresheners. Eat them liberally.

Keep handy a small bowl of whole cinnamon bark pieces, cloves, fennel seeds, and peeled cardamom pods to chew, for an alluring flavor your lover will want to kiss. My favorite breath-freshening remedy is to suck on a whole clove; it is long lasting and inexpensive. Even if you take a few bites of food, you can tuck the clove between your cheek and gum with your tongue and then bring it back in your mouth after eating.

Use acidophilus as a supplement if you suffer from bad breath. If you do eat garlic, get all your friends to eat it too, so no one will notice your garlic breath. Enjoy garlic at night when you will be in for the evening and not subjecting others to its smell. Eat a sprig of parsley or a small piece of lemon peel to freshen your breath. Drink a cup of peppermint tea or add two drops of anise, fennel, or peppermint essential oil to a glass of water before drinking.

Any of the following herbs can be made into a tea and used as a breath-freshening mouthwash: basil, chocolate mint, fennel, juniper berries, lavender flowers, parsley, peppermint, pineapple sage flowers, rose petals, sage, or thyme.

Fresh Breath Mouthwash

It is so easy to make an instant breath freshener!

1/2 cup water

4 drops anise, cinnamon, fennel, peppermint, or tea tree essential oil

Combine the ingredients in a cup. Swish, don't swallow, then spit.

CHIN AND NECK BEAUTY

The neck is a passageway for the central nervous system. It is said to be the place where we hold our will, and a flexible or rigid neck can affect our emotional countenance. The neck is one of the first parts of the body to show aging. Anger can be stored in the temporomandibular joints (TMJs) of the jaw. The three factors that can cause a double chin are anatomy, body fat, and time. Even some thin people can have double chins. When the skin loses some of its elasticity, parts of the body may sag. Lose weight. A hairstyle above the jawline will be the most flattering. Highlight other features with makeup, such as the eyes. Wear open, broad necklines. Avoid turtlenecks. As far as jewelry, wear longer necklaces and shorter or post earrings, as chokers and long dangling earrings will draw attention to the neck.

Chant. Sing. Be joyful. Share the love.

Remember to moisturize it using light oils, tapping gently to prevent a double chin. When moisturizing the neck, use gentle upward strokes starting from the base of the neck and working to the chin point.

Practice gentle neck rolls by dropping your chin to your chest and slowly moving your head clockwise three or four times and then counterclockwise. To strengthen your neck muscles, sit comfortably. Lean your head back and look toward the ceiling. Open your mouth, and to a count of five, bring your lower jaw up until your upper teeth rest inside your lower teeth. Hold for a count of five. Repeat two more times.

Make a neck mask by peeling and mashing a large tomato, and applying the pulp to your neck for an hour. Rinse off. Elder flower water is a traditional application to keep the neck from getting flabby and wrinkled. Apply it to your neck after bathing.

The Turtle is a Taoist exercise for the neck. Simply inhale while touching your chin to your chest, feeling the stretch on your shoulders and back of your neck. Then bring your shoulders up to your ears, like a turtle going into its shell. Exhale as you drop your head back to rest on the back of your neck, while practicing Kegel exercises (see page 136). Repeat twelve times.

NATURAL DEODORANTS AND FRAGRANCES

Natural Deodorants

Years ago, I had a wise older woman friend who told me she would never use commercial deodorants, as she believed they contribute to breast cancer. I thought that was ridiculous in my sixteen-year-old naïveté. Our government would never allow that! A few weeks later, while at boarding school, a bottle of the leading antiperspirant fell, smashing behind my dresser. The bell rang and I had to run off to class. Being a sloppy kid, it was a few days before I cleaned behind the dresser; I was amazed that the deodorant had hardened into a plasticlike sheet. I never bought commercial deodorant after that and instead only used what was aluminum free and as natural as possible from the health food store. Let your breasts and underarm lymph channels have free-flowing *chi*!

When our bodies are healthy, body odor should be pleasant and convey information about our hormonal and pheromonal state. Fresh perspiration is usually odorless, but when mixed with bacteria, it can take on a less savory hue.

To smell sweeter, clean up your body. Eat plenty of greens and drink lemon in water. Use super green foods like wheatgrass, spirulina, and barley grass. Take one to three chlorophyll capsules daily.

Harem women knew how to make themselves more alluring; they ate fenugreek seeds so they would exude a seductive smell. You could eat fenugreek sprouts or make a tea of this herb. My friend Herbal Ed always smells like amber, which creates its own kind of allure.

Many deodorants contain aluminum chlorohydrate, a man-made form of aluminum that is linked to Alzheimer's disease. It is known to accumulate in the tissues, especially when applied to broken skin. (Yikes! This is often done after shaving.) Many deodorants also contain synthetic fragrances and methyl- and propylparabens, both of which have been implicated in breast cancer. Look for deodorants that contain natural ingredients, such as coriander and tea tree oil. You can find some good deodorants in natural food stores. Weleda brand spray deodorants work great.

The exocrine glands (also known as the eccrine glands) are responsible for secreting the fluid known as sweat through a duct that moisturizes the skin, maintaining a healthy acid balance, and preventing unhealthy proliferations of microbes. It is the apocrine glands that secrete body odor. These glands occur throughout the body, including the armpits, face, chest, pubic, and anal regions. A person's scent will vary according to conditions of health and mental well-being. Blondes tend to have a more cheesy, sour natural body odor; brunettes tend to have a sweet, pungent type of perspiration; and redheads are more acrid and sharp in fragrance.

Sweat is made up of water, sodium salts, lactic acid, sulfuric acid, potassium, phosphorus, iron, and urea. It is normal to excrete between 1.7 and 2.6 pints of water each twenty-four hour period, though this amount can be up to ten times higher under conditions that cause perspiration. Factors that will increase perspiration include heat, exercise, hot spicy food, and stress.

Perspiration is supposed to leave the body, so preventing this can be a problem. A safe approach is to apply plain baking soda, cornstarch, or cosmetic clay to help prevent and absorb mild to moderate perspiration. Rub lemon peel (not the juice) or fresh sage leaves on dry skin to inhibit bacteria and odor. Aloe vera juice can be applied directly as an antibacterial, antifungal, and deodorizing ally.

Wise Witch Hazel Deodorant

Effective and cost effective!

1 ounce witch hazel

10 drops lavender essential oil or other essential oil of your choice

Combine the witch hazel and essential oil in a fine-spray mister bottle. Alternatively, store it in a glass bottle and apply it with a cotton ball.

Baking Soda Deodorant

This is for those who prefer a dry deodorant.

1 cup baking soda or white clay

30 drops lavender essential oil

20 drops coriander essential oil

10 drops tea tree essential oil

Combine the baking soda and essential oils. Mix well. Store in a glass jar. Apply a dusting to the underarm area.

Be Sure You're Sure Deodorant

It's so easy to prepare this.

1/4 cup apple cider vinegar or vodka
1/4 cup distilled water
50 drops coriander essential oil or other essential oil of your choice

Combine the vinegar, distilled water, and essential oil in a fine-spray mister bottle. Alternatively, store it in a glass bottle and apply it with a cotton ball.

Deodoraroma

Essential oils are antibacterial and keep you smelling fresh.

3 tablespoons witch hazel
3 tablespoons distilled water
2 drops sage essential oil
2 drops lemon essential oil
2 drops tea tree essential oil
2 drops lavender essential oil

Combine the witch hazel, distilled water, and essential oils in a fine-spray mister bottle. Alternatively, store it in a glass bottle and apply it with a cotton ball.

Arrowroot Deodorant

This is a simple powder that really works.

6 tablespoons arrowroot powder
10 drops lavender essential oil
10 drops sage essential oil

Combine the arrowroot powder and essential oils. Mix well. Store in a glass jar. Apply a dusting to the underarm area.

Natural Fragrances

Rose Cologne

This is light and refreshing.

1 cup vodka
6 tablespoons rose water
1 teaspoon lavender essential oil

Combine all the ingredients in a clean glass jar.

Herbal Cologne

Make your own cologne in less than a minute.

- 2 cups vodka
- 1/4 cup water
- 1/4 teaspoon lemon essential oil
- 1/4 teaspoon neroli essential oil
- 10 drops rosemary essential oil

Combine all the ingredients in a clean glass jar and shake well. Apply to your pulse points, as you would use a perfume.

Floral Cologne

This is a traditional recipe.

- 1 cup water
- 1 cup vodka
- 2 tablespoons scented rose petals
- 2 tablespoons lavender flowers
- 1 teaspoon finely chopped orange peel
- 1 tablespoon rosemary leaves
- 1 tablespoon fresh spearmint leaves

Chop all the flowers and place in a glass jar with the water and orange peel. Cover with the vodka. Shake daily. Allow to steep for two weeks. Strain and press the oils out of the plants. Transfer to a clean glass bottle and store away from heat and light.

Simple Floral Water

- 100 ml (3.4 ounces) water
- 1–5 drops essential oil of your choice

Add the essential oil to the water and shake well.

Florida Water

"Florida" means "land of flowers." Use this as a refresher anytime.

- 2 cups vodka
- 1 1/2 teaspoons bergamot essential oil
- 1 teaspoon lavender essential oil
- 1/2 teaspoon clove essential oil
- 1/4 teaspoon lemon or lime essential oil

Combine all the ingredients in a clean glass jar.

Aphrodisiac Perfume

Love the one you're with.

16 drops rose or rosewood essential oil
8 drops jasmine essential oil
8 drops ylang-ylang essential oil
5 drops neroli essential oil
1 drop vanilla essential oil

Combine all the ingredients in a clean glass jar.

Lavender Water

Clean, fresh, and comforting.

1 cup fresh lavender flowers
1 cup vodka
1 cup distilled water

Cover the lavender flowers with the vodka. Cover, and allow to steep for two weeks. Strain and add the water. Store in a dark bottle away from heat and light.

Here are a few ideas for making simple natural perfumes. Just place a few drops of essential oil in a tiny clean glass bottle. Shake well. Apply to pulse points, such as behind the ears, wrists, and/or knees.

Floral Blend

15 drops rose essential oil
5 drops vanilla essential oil
1 drop jasmine essential oil

Herbal Blend

60 drops rosemary essential oil
40 drops lavender essential oil

Passion Potion

5 drops rose essential oil
3 drops ylang-ylang essential oil
3 drops jasmine essential oil

Exotic Blend

15 drops patchouli essential oil
20 drops sandalwood essential oil
5 drops rose essential oil

Woodsy Blend

50 drops pine essential oil
2 drops jasmine essential oil

CHAPTER 4

Beauty by Nature for Everyone

MEN'S BEAUTY

Men can benefit from most of the other sections in this book for health and beauty concerns. Here are just a few specifics for the bros.

Men's dermis (the lower skin layer) is thicker than women's due to hormones. Men tend to be more resilient from the damage of sun, wind, and cold. The collagen fibers in their dermis help keep the skin tighter. Yet they do wrinkle and need to take care of their skin and use moisturizer. Men who shave are exfoliating naturally.

I tell men who want to be more beautiful to delight in their own sensuality. Delight in colors, wear sensuous fabrics, and use pleasant-smelling products. Eat food that is super-charged with energy. Raw pumpkin seeds will help keep the prostate gland healthy.

Good fragrances for men include allspice, bay, cedarwood, coriander, fir, lime, mint, pine, rosemary, and sandalwood.

Easy Aromatherapy Aftershave

Here's a lovely way to make something with essential oils that really resonates with you.

2 cups distilled water

1/4 cup vodka or witch hazel

15 drops essential oil of your choice

Combine all the ingredients and store in a glass bottle. Splash on your face and neck as desired.

Bay Rum Aftershave

Used by pirates everywhere for centuries. Splash it on after shaving or whenever you want to feel invigorated.

- 2 cups rum
- 1/2 cup bay leaves
- 1/4 cup ground cloves
- 1/4 cup ground allspice berries
- 1/4 cup chopped fresh gingerroot

Cover the herbs with rum in a clean glass jar and allow to steep for two weeks. Strain out the herbs and store the remaining liquid in a glass bottle.

Island Aftershave

Nice and spicy!

- Juice of 2 fresh limes
- 1 cup witch hazel
- 15 drops lime essential oil
- 10 drops lavender essential oil
- 10 drops bay essential oil
- 1 cup rose water
- 1 teaspoon tincture of benzoin

Combine all the ingredients. Store in a clean glass jar.

Herbal Aftershave

Liven up yourself! Bob Marley would be proud.

- 2 cups witch hazel
- 1 tablespoon rosemary
- 1 tablespoon spearmint
- 1 cinnamon stick
- 7 whole cloves
- Peel from 1/2 orange
- Peel from 1 lime
- 15 drops tincture of benzoin

Place all the ingredients in a glass bottle and allow to steep for two weeks. Strain out the herbs and bottle the liquid. Splash on your face after shaving.

LOOKING GOOD WHEN YOU DON'T FEEL GREAT

We've all had those days. Up with a sick baby all night, or with our lover, making love (or war) till the wee hours of the morning. Ideally, you can get some rest, but there are those times when the day after a hard night has us facing an important presentation or interview. Here are a few tips to get you through the day. Even just doing a few of them can give positive results.

- Do three minutes of dry brush skin massage (see page 40).
- Take a shower with Dr. Bronner's peppermint soap. Use a facial scrub while in the shower. End your shower with cold water.
- Do a facial mask (see pages 33–37).
- Splash cold water (or snow) on your face or stick your face in the freezer for thirty seconds.
- Lie down for ten minutes (on a slant board if you have one) with cucumber slices (or a frozen gel mask) over your eyes.
- Do a yoga shoulderstand or headstand (only if you are adept at doing them).
- Drink a cup of water with lemon.
- Drink yerba maté tea during the day.
- Eat a crunchy green apple.
- Put your thumb in your mouth, push it high into the inside of your cheek cavity, and with the second and third fingers on the outside of your cheek, pull the skin away from your mouth, across to the ear, while pressing your cheekbone firmly. Repeat two to three times. This will give you a glow where you need it.
- Apply a bit of blusher and blue eyeliner.
- Take ten deep inhalations of lemon or peppermint essential oil. Do this several times daily.
- Use a natural citrus perfume.
- Do an exercise called Picking Grapes: Stand tall and reach high with one hand at a time, even getting on your tiptoes, to collect imaginary "grapes" from the ceiling. Breathe deeply while doing this.
- Wear loose but flattering clothing.

Voila! Hopefully tonight will be easier.

BABY BEAUTY

No doubt, babies are inherently beautiful! A gift from the universe. Children's hair is naturally beautiful and simple styles are best. A haircut is usually unnecessary until about age two.

Cradle Cap

Cradle cap is a type of infantile seborrheic dermatitis caused by overactive sebaceous glands, a natural buildup of cells, or in some cases a yeast called *Pityrosporum ovale*. It is not caused by poor hygiene. Babies may have thick, yellowish flaking of the skin and redness on the scalp, head, underarms, and groin area. It is not itchy, contagious, or painful, and tends to bother the parents more than the child. It usually begins between two weeks and three months of age and can last until the toddler stage.

At night, rub the baby's scalp with neem, olive, or sesame oil scented with a few drops of chamomile, lavender, rose, and rosemary or tea tree essential oils. Avoid using harsh soaps and shampoos on the baby. The baby's scalp can be washed with a tepid tea of burdock root, chamomile, chickweed, meadowsweet, or violet leaf. Leave the tea on the scalp; when it is dry, apply some coconut oil and rub it into the scalp to soften the crusts. Another remedy is to fill a cloth bag with uncooked rolled oats, wet the bag, and use the fluid that exudes from it to wash the scalp. Use a fine-tooth comb to loosen the afflicted spots. The nursing mom should include some flaxseeds and burdock root tea in her diet, as well as minimize dairy products, fried foods, and heated oils to help with fat metabolism.

Diaper Rash

Diaper rash may occur when the nursing mother's and/or baby's diet has become overly acidic. It may indicate that tomatoes, citrus products, sweets, or even fruits are being overconsumed or are aggravating the digestive system. Keep the baby's bottom diaper free as much as possible, and change the diapers more often. Avoid rubber or plastic pants as well as disposable diapers. If you launder your own cloth diapers, add one-quarter cup apple cider vinegar to the final rinse water. Expose the baby's bottom to fresh air by laying the child on an open, flat diaper, when possible, rather than fastening the diaper.

An application of plain yogurt to the baby's bottom may help to clear up a persistent diaper rash. Calendula salve can also be applied.

Consider giving the baby an acidophilus supplement internally that is formulated for infants. The nursing mother may also want to use an adult acidophilus internally. Acidophilus is a friendly bacteria that naturally occurs in yogurt.

Children's Teeth

It is best to keep babies from falling asleep while holding a bottle. When children sleep sucking bottles, the flow of saliva is decreased and sugars from milk or juice pool around the teeth, contributing to decay. Of course breastfeeding is the ultimate gift to bestow to your child.

As teeth develop, parents can wipe their children's gums and budding teeth with a clean washcloth. When the teeth have fully come in, parents can brush them until the children learn to do it properly themselves. Even then, you may want to brush over them while exclaiming what a great job they have done. A child's first visit to the dentist should be around age three.

LIVING A LONG AND HEALTHY LIFE

Beauty by Nature is filled with ideas on looking and feeling good for all of your life. This chapter focuses just a little extra on the concerns of the elderly.

Older skin consists of only two or three layers; thus it retains moisture less effectively. As we age, the skin becomes thinner, fewer cells are produced, and skin cells grow more slowly. Blood vessels become fewer, and sweat and oil gland activity decreases, which can make us more prone to itchiness and dryness. Collagen and elastin fibers become more rigid, leading to sagging and wrinkling.

Pick up the skin on the back of your hand with two fingers. Pull it gently and see how long it takes to return to its normal position. Snapping back is a sign of youthfulness. If it takes a long time, it is a sign of aging. You can learn to reverse the process. There is not a cell in the human body, except for in the teeth and bones, that is over eleven months old.

Avoid programming yourself with negative thoughts and expressions about aging, such as, "You can't teach an old dog new tricks," or "I'm not getting any younger." These are self-limiting affirmations. Let them go. They really aren't true. I don't know about your dog, but you can certainly feel younger and learn new tricks.

In the Asian tradition, it is believed that our vitality is depleted by stress and struggle. Wise people control their life force (*chi*) through skillful and easy action. Having a healthy attitude that includes living in the moment rather than fretting about the past or future is something positive to attain. The mind is the most important factor in how we age. When the mind is focused on negativity, age will overcome us more quickly. Embrace what is new, bringing the value of past lessons into the present moment.

If you use prescription drugs, avoid mixing them with alcohol. Never use someone else's prescriptions, and don't exceed the recommended dosage. Make sure your physician is aware of any other substances you are taking, including herbs, vitamins, and other prescription and nonprescription drugs. Remember that specialists filter your ailments through their expertise. Your chiropractor might feel your headaches are due to pinched nerves, while a neurologist might want to investigate a brain tumor. In truth, you might need to cut back on coffee.

Remember to count your blessings and be thankful for the many ways our bodies serve us. Rather than identifying too heavily with your health concerns (my arthritis, my hemorrhoids), make a list and give thanks for all of the wonderful ways your body does serve you. For example: I am grateful for my eyes that see the joy on my grandchildren's faces; I am grateful for my good hearing that allows me to listen to music and the comforting sound of my partner's voice.

You may find that the addition of the following substances can improve the quality and perhaps the length of your life.

- **Alfalfa** contains eight different digestive enzymes. It helps to regulate the pH of the stomach, thus improving digestion in people prone to acidity.
- **Ashwagandha** improves memory and facilitates learning. It also invigorates sexual *chi*.
- **Astragalus** strengthens the immune system, making us more resistant to disease.
- **Burdock root** helps the body eliminate excess uric acid, which may benefit some types of arthritis and gout and improves dry skin conditions.
- **Eleuthero** increases endurance and helps the body acclimate to mental and physical stress.
- **Garlic** helps to prevent blood platelets from clumping together. It also lowers triglycerides and reduces bad cholesterol.
- **Ginger** is well known for its ability to relieve nausea and digestive distress. It also helps to improve circulation to the extremities and aids in pain relief from arthritis. Much like aspirin, yet without the side effects,

ginger inhibits blood platelet aggregation and therefore is useful in preventing strokes and heart failure.

- **Ginkgo** helps the brain to better utilize oxygen and glucose.
- **Ginseng** improves energy levels and enhances mental alertness. It also has immune-strengthening benefits. It is able to lower harmful LDL cholesterol while increasing beneficial HDL cholesterol.
- **Hawthorn berries, leaves, and flowers** help to dilate the blood vessels, thereby lowering blood pressure. They are naturally high in flavonoids, thus strengthening the capillaries. They also improve the contraction force of the heart and our utilization of oxygen.
- **Ho shou wu** is both a kidney and liver tonic. It is used to enhance libido, increase energy, and promote hair health.
- **Jujube dates** are a sedative and cardiotonic. They help to relax smooth muscles and are considered a tonic for the nervous system. In Asian medicine, jujube is used for weakness, shortness of breath, and irritability.
- **Licorice root**, in Asian medicine, is known as "the great harmonizer" and is often added to herbal formulas. It is an excellent anti-inflammatory agent, helps to speed the healing of ulcers, and is supportive to the adrenal glands. Licorice can improve energy levels and muscle tone. Those with high blood pressure or edema should consult with a competent health professional before using licorice internally for extended periods.
- **Lycii berries** are used in Asian medicine to help promote cheerfulness and a long life. They improve vitality and vision.
- **Milk thistle seeds** contain three types of flavonoid molecules that work as antioxidants and have a strong affinity for the liver.
- **Milky oat seeds** are rich in bone-building minerals and are calming to the nerves.
- **Nettle** is a highly nutritious herb that is particularly strengthening to the kidneys and builds the blood.
- **Reishi mushrooms** are used in Asia, where they are regarded as a symbol of youth and longevity. Reishi is even called "the plant of immortality."
- **Green tea leaves** are an antioxidant that aid in fat metabolism and reduce the risk of arterial disease.

These herbs are often available in various combinations and may be used as teas, tinctures, or in capsules. Chinese patent formulas are widely available in stores that sell Asian herbs. See what is available at your local natural food store. Rejuvenating essential oils include frankincense, lavender, myrrh, neroli, rose, and tea tree.

THE TIBETAN FIVE RITES

There are several books and videos available that extol the virtues of the Tibetan Five Rites, a series of exercises practiced by Tibetan lamas, who are known for their longevity. I find the exercises simple, wonderful for aligning the back and neck, invigorating for the endocrine system, and helpful for improving the flow of energy in the body. They are said to slow down the aging process. You will need a clean, open space on a rug, mat, or floor. Start doing each exercise seven times; within a few weeks, work up to doing each rite twenty-one times. If you are sick, stressed, or too busy, do each rite just three or so times rather than skipping them altogether. The best approach is to do the rites first thing in the morning on an empty stomach.

The First Rite

This one involves simply spinning clockwise (up to twenty-one times) with your arms held out to your sides (your right arm leads). To prevent dizziness, fix your gaze on a stationary object at eye level in the room, such as a painting. Lie down on your back on the floor immediately afterward, bring your hands above your head, and breathe and

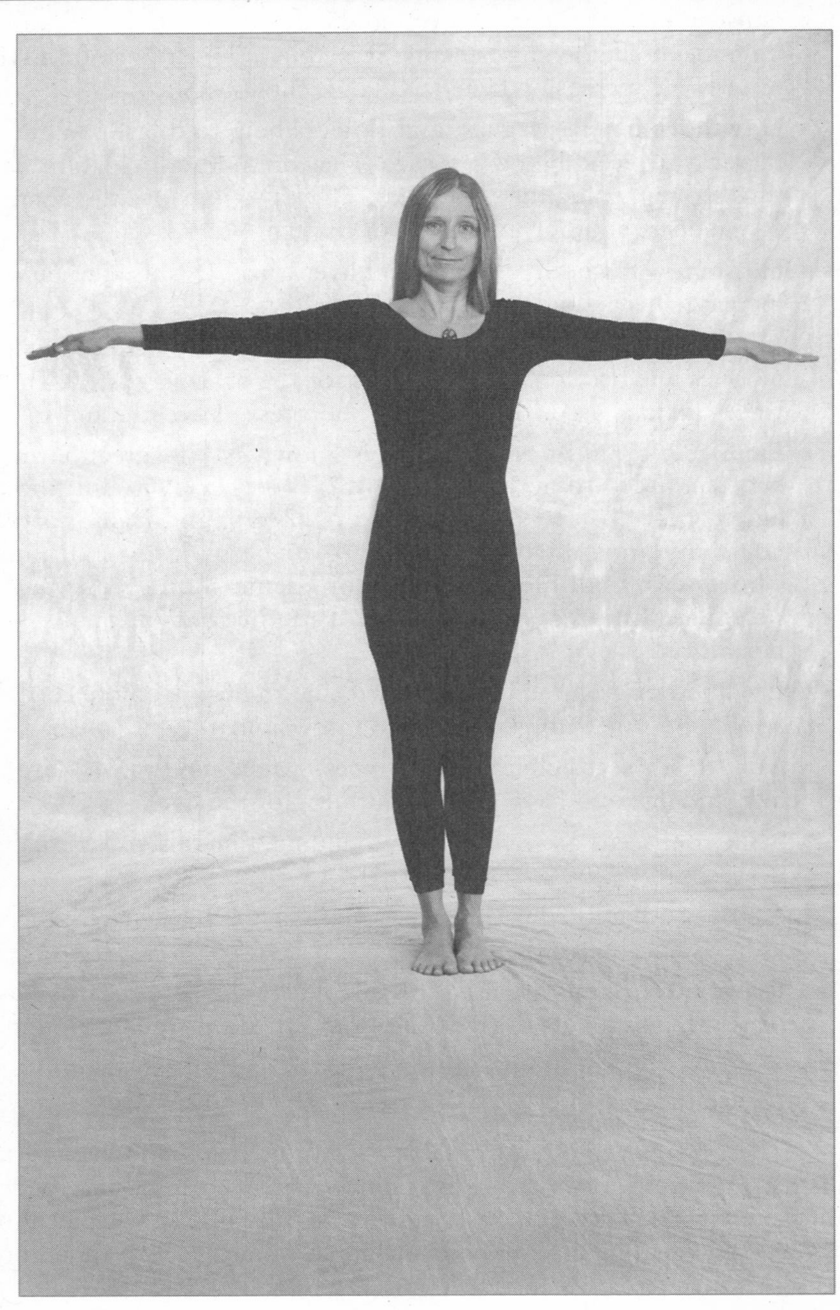

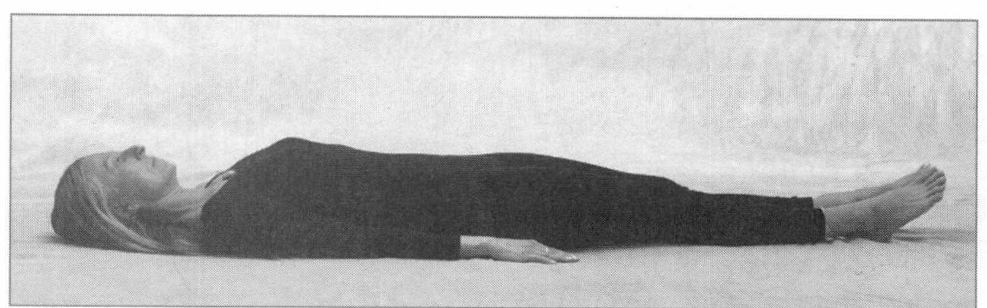

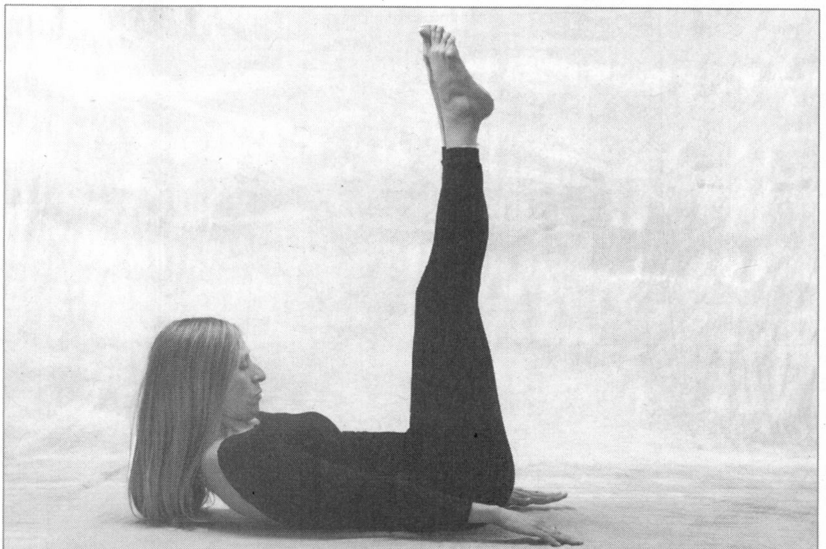

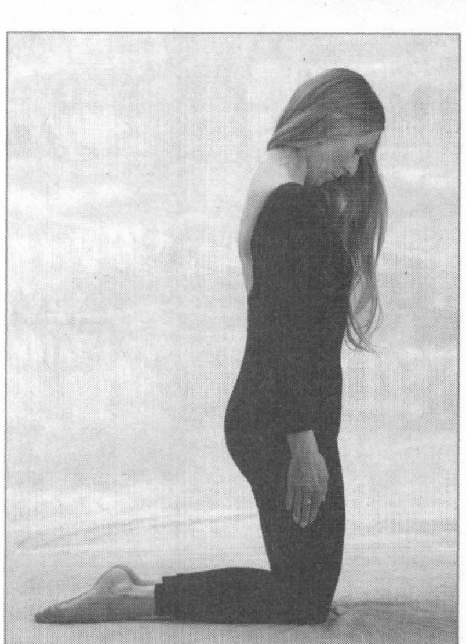

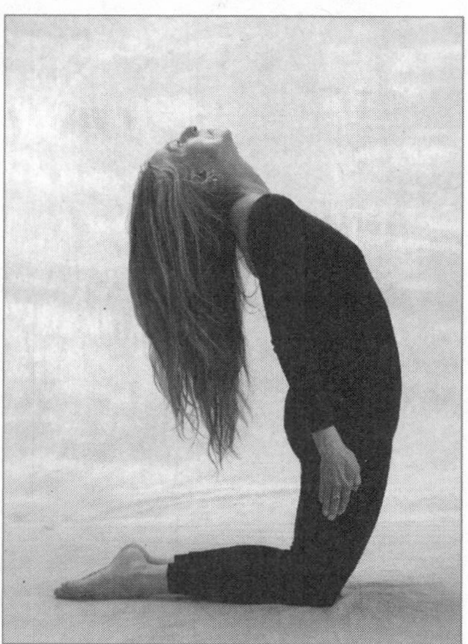

stretch your body. The spinning exercise helps relieve varicosities, strengthens digestion, improves brain function, and can even cast off negative energies. Allow any dizziness to pass before continuing to the second rite.

The Second Rite

Lie on your back on the floor. Press into the floor with your forearms, elbows, and shoulders. Tuck your chin to your chest as you inhale and lift both legs toward your head. Keep your abdomen pulled in. Exhale and slowly lower your legs. Relax. Repeat up to twenty-one times. The second rite has a restorative effect on the thyroid, adrenals, kidneys, and sex and digestive organs.

The Third Rite

The third rite is done by kneeling on the floor. Place your hands beside your thighs. Exhale and lower your chin to your chest. As you inhale, close your eyes and lean back while fully arching your back. Return to the original position. Repeat up to twenty-one times. The third rite helps balance the neck, back, heart, lungs, thyroid gland, sinuses, and digestion.

The Fourth Rite

The fourth rite begins in a seated position, with your legs stretched out in front and your hands at your sides. Exhale as you touch your chin to your chest. With concentrated strength, inhale and raise your head all the way back while lifting your body horizontally to the floor by pushing with your feet and hands, as if you were trying to become a table. Keep your buttocks tight to avoid placing stress on your lower back. Sweep back down to the original sitting position. This exercise benefits arthritis, osteoporosis, irregular menses, and sinus congestion.

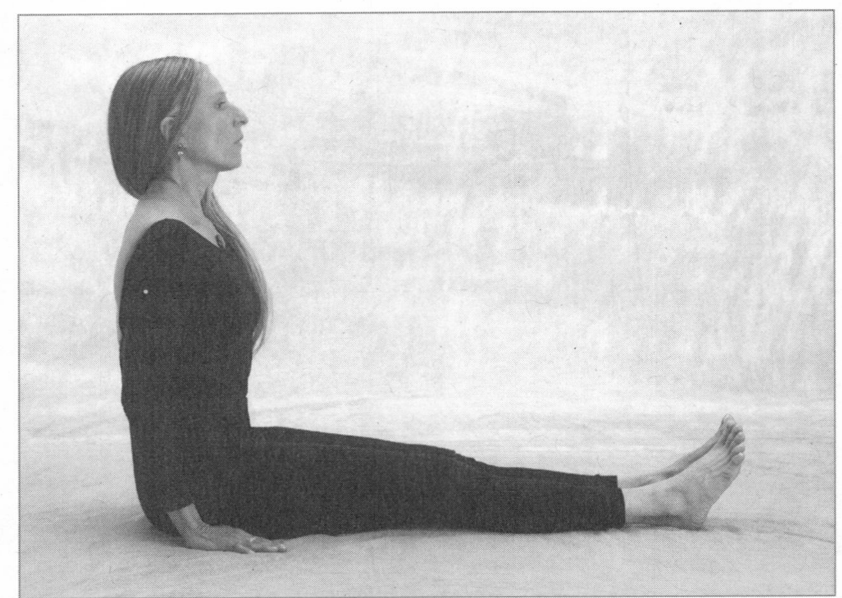

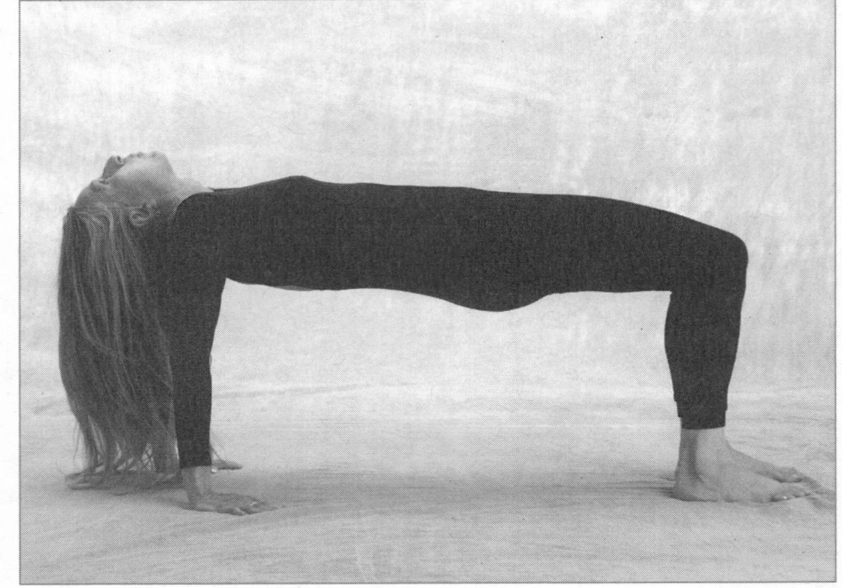

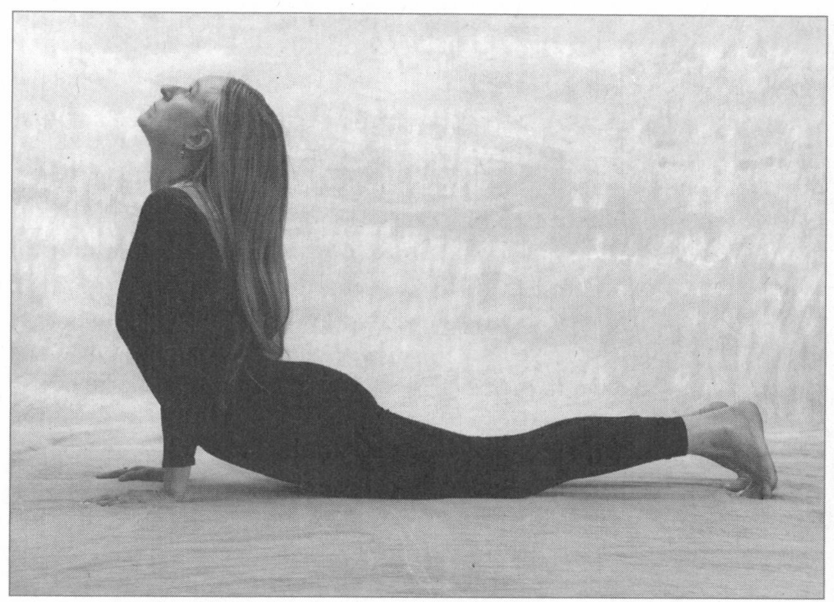

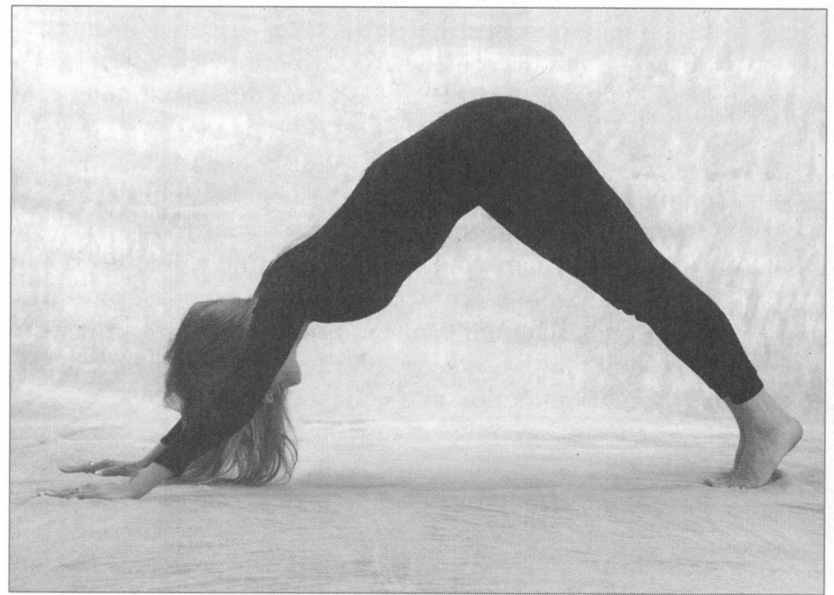

The Fifth Rite

The fifth rite begins as if you were about to do a push-up. Lie face down on the floor, your arms and legs supporting you, and your legs spread straight out, about shoulder width apart. Exhale and bring your head back and arch your body into a sagging position. Inhale, tuck in your chin, and bend at your hips, making a pyramid-like shape. Exhale and sweep again into the first position. Repeat up to twenty-one times. This portion of the Five Rites benefits arthritis, osteoporosis, sinus congestion, back pain, digestive and bowel concerns, and leg and neck stiffness.

It's ideal to rest five to ten minutes after completing the rites. Lie on your back with your eyes closed.

Drinking Water

May you never thirst.

—STARHAWK, *THE FIFTH SACRED THING*

Water rejuvenates the cells, facilitates the digestive and eliminative processes, carries nutrients to the body's tissues, helps rid the body of toxins, maintains body temperature, aids in pH balance, and provides liquid for cells. Drinking water bathes the internal organs, aids respiration, stimulates kidney function, dilutes bodily fluids, and provides energy and nourishment. It also moistens the skin, helps purify the blood, diminishes allergies, reduces the growth of yeasts, slows aging, and flushes out contaminants, toxins, and bacteria.

Drink water first thing in the morning. I love to make cold water infusions with fresh blossoms, such as lilacs, organic rose petals, or violets, or with fresh herbs, such as lemon balm or spearmint. This is done by simply putting a couple of handfuls of blossoms or herbs into a jar and covering them with water. Allow the mixture to sit at room temperature for about three hours, and then enjoy a beauteous herbal-infused drink. Try putting a slice of fresh lemon, lime, orange, or cucumber into water. You can even add crystals (too big to swallow) into water to energize it. Float flowers in water. Share your special water with others.

continued

FOOD FOR BEAUTY

Beauty ultimately comes from the inside. Food is one of the things we can control in our lives. Digested food ultimately becomes our blood. What do you choose to be composed of?

The right foods reduce puffiness and inflammation and promote a healthy-looking glow. Having worked in the fields of health and nutrition for over thirty-five years, I have seen a multitude of trends and diets come and go: high protein, low carbohydrate, high carbohydrate, vegan, vegetarian, high fat, low fat, macrobiotic, mucusless, and everything else you can imagine. Since 2000, I have eaten primarily a raw food diet consisting mostly of fresh fruits and vegetables and raw nuts and seeds. There are many delicious recipes featured in my book *Rawsome!* (Basic Health Publications, 2004).

Eating more healthfully is not only excellent for becoming your most beautiful self, but better health can also be your birthright. Moods become brighter. Bones become denser. Skin becomes more radiant. Immunity is revitalized.

Inflammation is at the root of poor health and rapid aging. All of the *–itis* diseases—such as cellulitis, colitis, bronchitis, and arthritis—can be reduced and improved with an enzyme-rich diet. Inflammation can also exist at a cellular level and can contribute to wrinkles, puffiness, bloatedness, and edema. Enzymes, which are present in raw food that has not been heated to over 114 degrees F, reduce inflammation and enhance beauty.

Cutting out refined sugars, grains, and even beans will help you be slimmer, have less facial puffiness, more beautiful skin, fewer wrinkles, improved skin coloring, and triumph over cravings and addictions. Alcohol will dehydrate your skin and hair. Caffeine can stimulate adrenaline production (which is involved in our "flight or fight" reaction), thus causing exhausted adrenal glands. Eating a food that you are allergic to can cause puffiness and inflammation. Dairy, wheat, corn, soy, eggs, sugar, and yeast are among the most common food allergens. Just because a food is organic doesn't mean it's healthful.

Organic macaroni and cheese in a box is still a highly processed food.

Fresh fruits and vegetables are rich in natural antioxidants, which can help prevent cellular damage and visible aging. Antioxidants prevent the formation of damaging free radical molecules, which are created when we are exposed to pollutants, smoke, heated oils, chemicals, and even food and water stored or served in plastic containers.

Here are a few reasons to check out a raw food diet, and if you choose to just eat more fresh fruits and vegetables and raw nuts and seeds rather than going 100 percent raw, you'll still benefit and beautify. Since I've been raw, I've had the clearest skin of my life; I can eat as much as I want and weigh what I want; and I have clear vision, boundless energy, and feel happier than ever. Even singing and dancing feel enhanced. I feel more fit now than I did twenty years ago.

For the uninitiated, going raw might seem like a daunting task. However, for those who make the raw transition, the benefits are many. A raw food diet may slow down the aging process. You may find that you feel better, have more energy, and need less sleep. Bad breath and body odor may be diminished. Many people report that they can normalize their weight without dieting. You may find that your eyes become brighter, your voice clearer, and your skin and muscle tone are improved.

The raw movement is the future. If it is possible to experience a higher state of consciousness, better health, more beauty, eat more delicious food, and save time and money, why not say yes to raw? If eating raw food could reverse the aging process and help you to be your most beautiful self, have clearer skin, attain your ideal weight, and get fewer wrinkles, why not say yes to the life force energy that flows from the sun to the harvest to you, Dear Beauty.

Live food infuses our being with fresh, vibrant energy, capable of resisting disease and helping us feel clear and bright. For some, a gradual transition is what feels right. Many find that the start of a new season (spring, summer, or fall) is a good time for new beginnings. Some people

I do not recommend drinking bubbly mineral water, unless it's the healthiest thing at a party. It contains carbon dioxide, which is something our bodies are actually trying to get rid of when we exhale; ingesting too much carbon dioxide can cause bloating and fluid retention.

Look for the best technologies in modern nontoxic purification methods, such as reverse osmosis systems, which are quiet and effective. Just be sure to change the filters as directed.

At the minimum, use a water filter in your showerhead; the filtered water can also be used to fill the bath. Even better, consider getting a whole-house water filter. Water is often purchased in plastic bottles, which can transfer petrochemicals into the water. Use glass whenever possible. I am delighted that in Boulder, Colorado, we can get mountain springwater delivered in glass bottles.

Water fluoridation is not something I agree with. Visit my Web site at www.brigittemars.com to read my article on water fluoridation.

Boiling water in a vaporizing chamber where steam rises and pollutants are removed makes distilled water. Distilled water is a neutral medium and has a magnetic attraction to unnecessary minerals in the body. Naturopaths recommend distilled water for arthritis and kidney stones, because of its absence of minerals. If you drink distilled water, consider taking a mineral supplement.

think that eating only raw food will be difficult. It isn't; it actually saves time, money, and our health. It's so worth it.

To stop eating familiar fare abruptly can be a shock to some people's systems. If slower transitions are more your style, start each meal with something raw, or make one meal a day raw. Have salad as the main dish rather than a side. Gradually increase the proportion of raw to cooked food. Try a new fruit or vegetable every week. Some people jump into raw 100 percent, and some are comfortable going fifty-fifty.

Eliminate heavier unhealthful foods that you know aren't good for you. If you must eat something cooked, steamed vegetables, amaranth, quinoa, millet, baked winter squashes, and baked sweet potatoes are the best choices. Bake or steam foods rather than fry them. Let go of packaged foods, instant fixes, frozen meals, and ready-to-eat, chemically tainted, and refined empty foods that damage health. If you overdo sugars, eat greens and fats for balance. Have cooked food at the end of the day; this will help you eat less of it. If you are cold, have miso soup or hot tea. Replace dairy products, eggs, and meat with avocados, nuts, and seeds. For some people, it can take a year to become totally raw. Eventually, remove all the cooked, canned, and processed food out of your cupboards. Increase raw food, and decrease cooked food. If you are still eating cooked food, eat more vegetarian meals, then eventually vegan meals. Replace cooked fats with raw fats. Shop at natural food stores or markets that sell organic produce. Select foods in season as much as possible. Eat only during daylight.

It's probably better to eat raw conventional produce than cooked organic produce. However, raw and organic is the ultimate. Only extended conditions of food shortage should cause us to eat food that is less than ideal. Start your day with a cup of warm water and the juice of half a fresh lemon. The sour flavor helps activate liver function, which in turn will encourage good bowel health and fat metabolism. Lemons in water help purify the body and provide mood-stabilizing lithium. Starting your day with stimulants (such as coffee) is like driving your car on a cold day without warming it up first. If I do need a stimulant, I prefer green tea or yerba maté. Although both of these contain some caffeine, they are also rich in antioxidants and less stressful on the adrenal glands.

An alternative to cooking is to "cook" without heat: marinate, ferment, or dehydrate. Using salt, oil, or lemon, and puréeing and drying are ways of making food look and taste more familiar without destroying the vitality of enzymes. Dehydrated dishes can take the place of cooked meals.

It is ideal to drink six or more glasses of water in the morning and then only have fruit until noon daily. Drink enough water during the day so that your urine is a pale golden color. Drinking at least two quarts of pure water a day is essential. Water helps to eliminate substances that would clog the pores. Fresh vegetable juices made with beets, celery, spinach, parsley, and cucumber will make your skin glow. Alcoholic beverages and caffeine-containing sodas and coffee can dehydrate your skin. A raw food diet is rich in living water (the water is not cooked out of the food), so you may not need to drink quite as much when eating mostly raw food. Equip your kitchen with a water purifier, juicer, blender, food processor, food dehydrator, and other practical tools that will make raw food preparation easier and more fun and versatile. Overeating even healthful food causes blood to be diverted to the stomach to aid digestion, thus leaving the skin lacking all it deserves.

Free radicals are unpaired molecules that quickly seek out another paired electron, thus causing free radical damage. Free radical damage, which occurs on an atomic level, can deteriorate the support structures of the skin, decreasing resiliency and elasticity. Antioxidants slow down free radical damage by preventing oxidative action of the free radicals. Eating a diet rich in antioxidants is the best defense against free radicals. Antioxidant nutrients include vitamins A, E, and C, the amino acids L-cysteine and methionine, the enzymes catalase and superoxide dismutase, and the coenzymes lipoic acid and Q10. Glutathione and methylsulfonylsulfate, commonly known as MSM, are also considered free radical scavengers. Many researchers believe that if indeed there is a fountain of youth, that antioxidants may be the answer. Of course, fresh fruits and vegetables are rich in antioxidants.

> Not everyone agrees on what is the best water to drink. In my home, we have a water filter that filters everything that comes out of the faucets, even for showers and baths. The filters get changed about twice a year. We do have a water distiller, though for drinking we get local springwater delivered in glass bottles. Water is referred to throughout this book. Use quality water for drinking and making beauty preparations. At the very least, use filtered water; better yet, use spring or distilled.

Get off of heated oils, which expose the body to free radicals, and use only unheated extra-virgin olive oil and raw coconut oil. Trans fats occur when oil is heated. Any time oil turns to smoke or food is browned, protein becomes a carcinogenic substance called acrolein. Trans fats have an adverse effect on the protective enzymes in the body that may be anti-inflammatory. Expeller pressed oils are usually heated, bleached, and deodorized. The protective polyphenols in olive oil are destroyed in cooking. Commercial salad dressings contain oils that have been heated.

Not all fats are bad, however. Healthful fats are found in foods like raw nuts and seeds, avocados, sun-cured olives, extra-virgin olive oil, and cold-pressed coconut oil. Our skin, hair, nails, hormones, digestive system, and nerves need quality fats to function properly.

Learn about organic flowers, such as hibiscus, rose, and violet. Make your food more beautiful, and entice your lover, family, and friends with the sacred designs of your presentations. Flowers are designed to attract pollinators and stream in color, design, and often fragrance. Be one with the flowers. “Flower power” always was a good idea. Let flowers fill your senses.

Use more antioxidant herbs and spices such as basil, coriander, cumin, dill, fennel, ginger, oregano, parsley, rosemary, sage, thyme, and turmeric. They are beautifying as well.

Beautifully Fresh Raw Foods

- Acai berries
- Almonds
- Apples
- Avocados
- Bananas
- Beets
- Berries
- Blueberries
- Burdock root
- Cabbages
- Cacao
- Camu-camu
- Cantaloupe
- Carrots (with the skin)
- Celery
- Cherries
- Coconut
- Coconut water
- Cucumbers
- Edible flowers
- Kale
- Limes
- Lucumas
- Maca
- Mangosteens
- Nuts, raw
- Papayas
- Parsley
- Perilla leaf
- Purple corn
- Radishes
- Red peppers
- Sea vegetables
- Seeds, raw (especially black sesame seeds)
- Spinach
- Spirulina
- Sprouts
- Strawberries
- Sweet potatoes
- Watermelon
- Winter squash
- Goji berries (also known as lycii berries)
- Grapefruits (especially red and pink varieties)
- Super green foods (this includes foods such as wheatgrass, barley grass, and spirulina that are enzyme rich and high in phytonutrients and detoxifying chlorophyll; their consumption can result in clearer skin, fresher breath, and faster healing)

Can you be beautiful if you are congested and constipated? Not for long! Fresh raw foods are beauty foods. In the box at the left are a few favorites from beauties around the globe. (To learn more about the specifics of some of these power plants, see pages 179–220).

A NATURAL APPROACH FOR HEALTHY WEIGHT

About 34 million Americans are at least 20 percent over their ideal weight, and this can contribute to a wide variety of problems including heart disease, diabetes, and lethargy. Select what is ideal for your body and don't be overly influenced by unhealthy images that fashion magazines promote.

Cravings are more likely to occur when we are hungry. When you crave sweets, choose a crunchy fruit, such as an apple. Craving sweets may be an indication that your body really needs more protein. A dose of bitter herbal tincture (available at natural products stores) can help dispel a craving for sweets. Craving salty foods like chips may indicate that you need minerals, such as those found in sea vegetables. When you crave fats, a daily tablespoon of hempseed oil provides beneficial essential fatty acids that can help emulsify fat. Most cravings will pass within a few minutes. Taking a few deep, slow breaths may help.

Chemical sweeteners can actually cause us to crave more sweets by upsetting our blood sugar levels.

Find ways other than food to nourish yourself. Consider the sensual delights of a warm bubble bath, a massage, reading a great novel, or walking in a beautiful environment. Make a list of all the alternative ways to bring nurturing enjoyment into your life, besides food, and start doing them.

Keep a journal of what you eat and drink for a week to gain insight about your diet and know what you really are consuming. Keep a weekly shopping list and stick with it. Avoid the aisles in the grocery store that have the foods that are not on your diet.

Too often mealtime is a rush and continuation of the stress in our daily lives. Before eating, serve yourself, rather than eating out of containers. Serve portions on plates and avoid country-style platters on the table. Sit down, relax, look at your food and say a blessing, or take a few deep breaths to help get calm. It takes the average person about twenty minutes for the brain to receive the message that the body is satisfied. Put the fork down between bites. Avoid eating while reading or watching TV. Some people find that using a smaller plate and a cocktail fork or chopsticks reminds them to appreciate each bite.

For centuries, slender people in cultures throughout the world have recognized that sea vegetables are an important source of nutrition. Their natural iodine content nourishes the thyroid gland, which governs metabolism, thus improving the rate at which our digestion functions. Kelp and dulse can be added to many dishes and can reduce the amount of salt used to flavor food.

Start meals with a salad. Consider having your entrée with salad rather than an empty carbohydrate, such as pasta, mashed potatoes, or white rice. Make lunch, rather than dinner, your main meal. We require more fuel at midday than at night. Right after dinner, floss and brush your teeth to discourage any more food consumption. If you must eat something, choose an apple or raw carrot.

Exercise is essential in any weight-loss program, as it warms the body, improves digestion, and helps produce endorphins to improve mental outlook. Take up a craft that keeps your hands busy and out of the pretzel bowl, such as knitting, sewing, woodworking, origami, beading, or embroidery.

There are a multitude of herbs that have been used to help weight loss and many ways to spice up meals with flavorful culinary herbs, tasty broths, salsas, Nama Shoyu tamari, fresh lemon or lime juice, or even flavored vinegars. Use more spicy condiments, such as cayenne, cinnamon, coriander, garlic, and ginger. They are warming, strengthen the spleen, improve circulation, and hasten metabolism and the burning of brown fat; thus they are referred to as thermogenic. Brown fat lies deep within the body and surrounds vital organs, such as the adrenals, kidneys, and heart; it is not storage fat.

Natural food stores carry herbal combinations in teas, capsules, and tablets. When used along with a good diet and exercise program, herbs can help you let go of unnecessary weight. Using herbs for weight loss in therapeutic dosages during pregnancy is not recommended.

Bless your food. If you must eat food that has a lower quality or has a lower vibrational level than what you are accustomed to, hold your hands over it and energize it; this way it will be more beneficial to you. Prepare food with love.

- Buy organic.
- Support local farmers.
- Visit the farmers' market.
- Grow a garden.
- Make your food beautiful.

Herbs for Weight Loss

- **Alfalfa** aids digestion and contains eight digestive enzymes. When your body is provided with all the necessary elements, you are less likely to crave food that is not needed.

- **Amla fruit** is an antioxidant, blood tonic, laxative, nutritive, and rejuvenative. Amla is reputed to make people feel lighter and to promote love, longevity, and good fortune. It increases lean body mass while reducing fat.

- **Burdock** improves the elimination of metabolic wastes through the liver, lymphatic system, large intestines, lungs, kidneys, and skin. It makes an excellent spring detox or fasting tea. Burdock stimulates bile production, thus enabling fat breakdown in the body.

- **Cayenne fruit** is high in beta-carotene and vitamin C. It causes the brain to secrete more endorphins. It is considered thermogenic, which means it can rev up metabolism and aid in weight loss.

- **Chickweed** has laxative, liver cleansing, and nutritive properties. Chickweed nourishes the *yin* fluids and dissolves plaque in the blood vessels and fatty deposits in the body. It reduces inflammation and clears toxins. Chickweed can be added to juices, salads, soups, and other dishes.

- **Cinnamon** is a circulatory stimulant and diuretic. It helps dry dampness in the body, is thermogenic, and promotes a rosy complexion.

- **Dandelion** is a blood purifier, which means it aids in the process of filtering and straining wastes from the bloodstream. Dandelion helps clear the body of old emotions, such as anger and fear, that can be stored in the liver and kidneys. It is an excellent herb for weight loss, as the root improves fat metabolism and the leaves are diuretic.

- **Fennel seeds** were eaten by Greek Olympic athletes so they would gain strength, not weight. Roman ladies ate fennel seeds to prevent weight gain. The seeds were eaten by the poor during the Middle Ages when they had nothing else, or during long church sermons or days of fasting to stave off hunger. Fennel seeds are delightfully sweet and help to curb the appetite by stabilizing blood sugar levels.

- **Flaxseeds** curb hunger due to their bulk; they also lubricate the colon and promote better bowel movements. Just eat one to two tablespoons of flaxseeds per day; chew them well or grind or soak them before eating. Be sure to consume plenty of fluids to aid this excellent bulk laxative. Better yet, learn to make flaxseed crackers.

- **Garcinia fruit** is thermogenic and has been used to treat obesity and curb hunger. Native to South Asia, this plant keeps the body from turning carbohydrates into fat by inhibiting the synthesis of fatty acids. It lowers the production of low-density lipoproteins and increases the production of glycogen. It contains hydroxycitric acid, similar to the citric acid found in oranges and grapefruits, which reduces appetite, stabilizes blood sugar levels, and enhances digestion. Garcinia also appears to improve the body's ability to burn calories.

- **Ginger** stimulates amylase concentration in the saliva and aids in the digestion of starches and fatty foods.

- **Green tea** is diuretic and thermogenic. Green tea prevents the blood from "clumping" and forming clots that can lead to stroke.

- **Guar gum** seeds and pods are laxative. Guar gum helps lower serum cholesterol levels and blood glucose levels. It slows down the absorption of carbohydrates. It tends to swell up in the digestive tract, causing a feeling of fullness and thus decreasing hunger. It is used in capsules.

- **Guggulu** is used as a rejuvenative, stimulant, and thyroid tonic. Guggulu contains phytosterols and helps lower the unfriendly low-density lipoprotein while elevating the beneficial high-density lipoprotein. It helps prevent blood platelet aggregation and breaks up already formed blood clots. Because it helps activate thyroid function by improving iodine assimilation, it may encourage weight loss. It stimulates circulation, promotes flexibility, and increases energy. Guggulu promotes bowel regularity and the secretion of digestive juices.

- **Gymnema** has long been used to treat obesity. *Gurmar*, a word derived from "gurmarin," a constituent of the leaves of this plant, means "sugar destroyer." When people chew some of this leaf and then eat some sugar, the sweet taste is eliminated in a few seconds. The molecules of the gymnemic acid fill the receptor sites for one to two hours, preventing the taste buds from being activated by the sugar molecules in food; it actually blocks sugar from being absorbed during digestion. Gymnema improves glucose utilization, enhances insulin production, and helps us overcome sugar addiction. It contains stigmasterol, betaine, and choline. If you are insulin dependent, consult with your physician before using gymnema, as your insulin medication may need to be adjusted.

- **Hawthorn** is used to treat obesity and calms the spirit. In Asian medicine, hawthorn is used more as a digestive aid, whereas in Western medicine, it is considered more of a heart tonic. Hawthorn can be used to strengthen the joint linings, collagen, and discs in the back, and to help us better retain a chiropractic adjustment.

- **Hoodia** tricks the brain into thinking we've eaten, as it makes us feel full. Studies show that it reduces interest in food, delays the time after eating before hunger sets in again, and promotes a sense of fullness more quickly. It contains a substance known as P57 that is believed to suppress the appetite by affecting the nerve cells that send glucose to the brain, causing us to feel satisfied. It is not a stimulant and has no known side effects.

- **Nettle** is used to improve acne, cellulite, and obesity. Nettle leaf and root tone and firm tissues, muscles, arteries, and skin. Nettle helps curb the appetite and cleanses toxins from the body. Since nettle is energizing, it helps motivate us to stay on a healthful diet.

- **Psyllium seeds** and the outer husk of the seeds are employed as a laxative and stool softener. They are traditionally used to treat constipation and obesity. Because they tend to swell and create a feeling of fullness, they can help curb appetite. Always use psyllium with plenty of liquids, otherwise it can *cause* constipation. Psyllium can dilute digestive enzymes, so it is best taken between meals, especially before bed or first thing upon rising, rather than with food.

- **Yerba maté** cleanses the blood; stimulates the mind, respiratory, and nervous systems; and decreases the appetite.

Aromatherapy for Weight Loss

Instead of eating sweets, smell the sweet aromas of anise, fennel, and spearmint essential oils to pleasure the brain and dispel unnecessary urges to eat. Bitter orange helps deter a desire for sweets. Essential oils that are good to use for massage when wanting to lose weight include cypress, juniper, and rosemary. Grapefruit essential oil helps those who eat when under pressure. Bergamot essential oil helps deter food addictions.

The flower essence cherry plum, one of the Bach Flower Remedies, is useful for those who tend to go on eating binges.

Vitamin Therapy for Weight Loss

As the body burns fats, metabolic waste products known as ketones and lipid peroxides are produced. Using an antioxidant vitamin (or drinking a raw green juice) can help keep the body healthy during this process. The B-complex vitamins and vitamin C, zinc, and calcium-magnesium can decrease sugar cravings. Taking 200 micrograms of glucose tolerance factor chromium (GTF chromium) can be very effective in keeping blood sugar levels stable; it helps insulin work more efficiently and keeps your mind off sweets. Chromium also has been found to decrease blood lipid levels. A maximum of five tablets can be taken throughout the day, if needed. Decrease this amount as needed once you have improved your diet.

L-glutamine can help satisfy the body's craving for sugar and refined carbohydrates. The amino acid L-glycine also helps to control sugar addiction. Both of these amino acids have a calming effect on the brain. L-phenylalanine also helps the brain feel satisfied. Both phenylalanine and tyrosine are thermogenic.

A daily supplement of essential fatty acids can actually help improve the body's metabolism of fat and reduce fat cravings. Lipoic acid helps protect the liver against toxins and is an antioxidant. Coenzyme Q10, also known as ubiquinone, is an antioxidant that improves the ability to metabolize fats. It is present in almost all cells, but its concentration tends to decline with age.

For Those Who Want to Gain Weight

People who have long been underweight often find that they finally can gain weight and achieve a healthier balance on a raw or mostly raw food diet. My husband gained weight, which really suited him. I lost and he gained, even though we both were eating relatively the same things.

Some people who begin a totally raw diet become thin enough to concern their family and friends. Though this may happen initially, most people are usually able to gain back some weight, and it is typically better quality weight. Foods that can help you gain weight include avocados, bananas, dried fruits, pumpkin seeds, sunflower seeds, and nut butters. Have an extra smoothie or two during the day, and include some of these richer foods along with your regular meals. Eventually your weight should find its balance.

Choosing to lose weight can be an opportunity to pay more attention to yourself and improve your overall health. Losing half a pound per week is considered safe. Set goals for yourself. Make this an opportunity to live a healthful lifestyle that can add years and joy to your life. May you reveal your most beautiful self ever!

Weight Gain Smoothie

Add one or two of these a day to your regular meals to increase weight gain.

2 cups raw almond milk

1½ ripe bananas

3 pitted dates, soaked 20 minutes

1 tablespoon raw tahini

Combine all the ingredients in a blender and process until smooth.

C H A P T E R 5

Beauty by Nature Ingredients

PREPARATIONS

When buying herbs, select those that are colorful and fragrant in bulk and store them in glass jars away from light and heat. Purchase cut herbs rather than powdered, as powdering causes them to lose essential oils more quickly.

Keep a recipe file. When a recipe calls for "parts" rather than an amount, this is measured in weight, not quantity. Make small batches the first time around. No fancy equipment makes up for poor-quality herbs. Avoid aluminum and copper in all the equipment you use.

Label each mixture with the ingredients, how to use, whether it is for internal or external use, and the date it was made. You may want to have a separate grinder, such as a coffee grinder, that you use just for herbs. If you ever need to grind resinous or sticky herbs, place them in a freezer for a few hours first and they will shatter easily in a blender. It also helps if you put the blender or grinder in the freezer, too. When making herbal products, singing, praying, and blessings are always a good thing to add to your product!

Herbal Teas

Herb teas are soothing and warming. They give us the opportunity to taste the many flavors of plants, and this stimulates various actions. Tea also forces us to take time out of our busy days to sip and savor and take in. We can nourish our entire being.

Buying herbs in packaged tea bags means they have been powdered in a way that causes a more rapid loss of essential oils. If using fresh herbs (undried), double the amount of herbs. Return your herbs to the earth by adding them to your compost or garden!

Hot Infusions

This is also known as a tisane.

1 cup water
1 heaping teaspoon dried herbs (leaves and flowers)

Bring the water to a boil in a nonaluminum pot and remove from the heat. Add the herbs, stir, and cover. Let sit for at least 10 minutes. Strain.

Cold Infusions

2 cups cold water
4 teaspoons dried herbs (leaves and flowers)

Combine the water and herbs in a glass jar or bowl and let soak overnight. Strain and heat to drinking temperature if desired.

Decoctions

Decoctions are used for roots and barks. If a root is particularly high in volatile oils (such as ginger or valerian), it is best infused rather than boiled. Some roots can be used a second time.

1 cup water
1 heaping teaspoon dried herbs (roots and bark)

Combine the water and herbs in a nonaluminum pot. Bring to a low boil, cover, and simmer for 20 minutes. Strain.

Sun Tea

You can also make sun tea or moon tea for that matter! Place the herbs in a jar for sun tea, or in an open glass bowl for moon tea. Let the herbs and water sit outside and collect the radiant energy. Drink moon tea first thing in the morning.

Overnight Jar Method

This is my favorite method for making a truly remedial tea. This process is excellent for extracting the maximum amount of medicinal potential from an herb. It takes time, but it is well worth the effort. Add about two ounces of roots or bark or one ounce of flowers or leaves to the bottom of a clean canning jar. Cover with boiling water and put the lid on. Allow the herbs to steep for as long as thirty minutes for seeds, two hours for flowers, four hours for leaves, and overnight for roots or bark. In the morning, strain the herbs out and enjoy the nutrient-rich brew. This method is not suggested for licorice root, slippery elm bark, or valerian root, as these will simply taste too medicinal or, in the case of slippery elm, become too mucilaginous to bear consuming.

Herbal Oil

Make sure all your equipment is dry (jars, lids, spoons, etc.), as moisture can cause mold and spoilage. Use dried herbs or wilt fresh herbs; the only exception is St. John's wort oil, which should be made from the fresh plant. Place the freshly crushed herbs in a glass jar and cover with olive oil. Be sure all the herbs are submerged under the oil, and add more, if necessary, if the plant expands. Top it off with more oil to discourage bacterial growth. Avoid having a large air space at the top of the jar. If bubbles appear in the oil while it is steeping, don't be alarmed; this is caused by gases in the herbs and doesn't indicate spoilage.

Oil may collect under the lid and seep out, creating a mess, so place a dish or pan under the jar to catch any leaks. I prefer to place some cheesecloth and a rubber band around the top of the jar, rather than using a jar lid, so any moisture can evaporate.

Put the jar of herbs and oil in a pan of hot water in the oven. Leave it in the oven for several hours with the heat turned to the lowest setting. In European herb lore, jars are sometimes placed in the sand (or even in a sandbox) to attract heat and allowed to become infused with earth energies for a couple of weeks. Some people like to put the oils in the sun, but this can increase the likelihood of spoilage.

Next, strain out the herbs. This can be done by lining a stainless steel strainer or a potato ricer with clean muslin and pouring in the oil and herbs. The oil obtained from pressing the herbs should be kept separate from the oil poured through the strainer, as it has more water in it and should be used up first (water can encourage spoilage). If herbal oils are stored in the sun, they can go rancid. Storing herbal oils in the refrigerator will help them to last from several months to several years.

Dosages

For Herbs

Herbs can be powdered in a blender and put in capsules. Natural food stores offer empty gelatin and vegetarian capsules that can be filled. This can be done by hand, or you can find many hand "machines" that will cap about fifty at once.

In general, one cup of tea equals one dropperful of tincture or two capsules or tablets. If dealing with an acute condition, such as fighting an infection, it may be necessary to use either one cup of tea, a dropperful of tincture, or two capsules or tablets every two waking hours, at least for a few days. As the condition improves, make those dosages further apart.

For Homeopathic Remedies

Usually four pellets are placed under the tongue and allowed to dissolve there. It is best to not eat or drink anything for ten minutes before or after taking the remedy. Some homeopaths recommend avoiding coffee, mint, and camphor while using homeopathic remedies.

For Vitamins

Check the label for dosage suggestions.

For Children

Take the child's approximate weight and divide by 150. For example, a fifty-pound child would take one-third of the adult dose.

MATERIA MEDICA

Beauty Ingredients

Natural cosmetics and other beauty aids have been used by millions of people for thousands of years. They have been time tested. We don't need to test them on rabbits or monkeys to see how much it takes to make 50 percent of them go blind or die. However, just because a substance is natural does not mean that someone can't have a reaction to it. Poison ivy is completely natural.

"Natural" means that the product ingredients were derived from plant or other organic materials and not synthesized. Natural skin care products may only contain a small percentage of natural ingredients. Don't be seduced by labels proclaiming that products are natural but really aren't. The Food and Drug Administration (FDA) does not regulate these claims.

Enzymes are often touted as ingredients in natural cosmetics, but they do deteriorate quickly. "Noncomedogenic" means the product is unlikely to cause the skin to break out. "Hypoallergenic" means that the product is less likely to cause an allergic reaction or sensitivity. However, people can be allergic to almost anything, including natural products. Just because a product is labeled hypoallergenic doesn't mean that it is natural or safe for everyone to use. Doing a personal patch test can be helpful. If you are allergic to something taken internally, such as chamomile or mangoes, it might cause an allergic reaction (such as a rash) when used topically. People with very sensitive skin should do a patch test on their forearm. To do this, apply a bit of the product to the inside of your forearm. If you are testing an essential oil, dilute one drop of oil with one tablespoon of water, and apply it with a cotton ball to the same area. Place a Band-Aid over the product you are testing and leave it on for twenty-four hours. Remove the Band-Aid and observe your skin. Any redness or rash can indicate an allergy. If swelling or irritation develops, don't use the product.

Some skin reactions to a particular product don't happen immediately. Over time we can become more sensitive. Also, a combination of factors can be implicated in a sensitivity. Of course, always consider what you have been eating that might have contributed to a skin problem. If you experience an allergic reaction, avoid using the product again, allow your skin to breathe, minimize sun exposure, and drink plenty of water. Dandelion root and/or nettle tea can help the body get rid of irritants. Take note of what might have been the cause of the reaction. Replace the cosmetic with another product after the irritation has cleared up.

Storing Your Natural Products

Blue or amber glass bottles are most excellent for storing homemade natural products, as they keep out excess light, thus increasing a product's shelf life. Wide-mouth jars make it easier to get the product out, especially for creams and salves, which don't pour easily. Metals tend to react with some substances and are not ideal for storing body care products. When using recycled jars to make your own cosmetics, always remove the inner cardboard lid, which can be a breeding ground for bacteria. When putting a lid down from a cosmetic product, place it upside down, so it is less likely to pick up dirt, hair, or other contaminants that can cause products to spoil. Wash your hands before dipping into products or ingredients; better yet, pour the product into your hand or use a clean spoon, spatula, swab, or cotton ball. Take out only what is needed, to avoid contaminating the rest of the container.

Be sure to label all your homemade skin care products, including how they are to be used. (I wonder how many people have swallowed suppositories they assumed were to be used as a pill?) Use permanent markers and cover the label with clear tape, so the writing can't be rubbed off by handling.

Store all cosmetics away from heat and light. When making natural cosmetics, it is imperative that you work with clean hands and utensils. Make small batches and refrigerate what isn't being used. Use up the product within a few weeks, and then make a fresh batch. You can keep makeup and moisturizers in the fridge. Products will last several months if kept in the fridge rather than in a hot, steamy bathroom. In general, store cosmetics in clean, dry, airtight containers. Water contamination can encourage the growth of unfriendly microorganisms. Any moist homemade products are best refrigerated. Products made from fresh fruits and vegetables usually last just one day; after that they should be composted. (I like to return things to the Earth Mother.)

Products that do not contain water (such as lip balms and salves) usually last at least a year when stored at room temperature, or longer if refrigerated. Most alcohol-containing products (such as some sprays, deodorants, and colognes) will last up to a year. Most homemade shampoos will keep for a week. Be sure to select only cold-pressed oils that are free of preservatives, and store them in the refrigerator to preserve their freshness. "Cold pressed" means that the products were extracted mechanically, usually at temperatures under 125 degrees F.

One of the keys to having oil-and-water-based products emulsify is to have all the ingredients at room temperature.

If a product separates, don't worry; just stir the ingredients back together with a clean utensil. Keeping products refrigerated will help decrease the likelihood of separation. Just keep enough product in the bathroom to last you a few days. Shake your natural products before using them. If something smells bad, grows mold, or changes color, it is best to throw it out. Do not heat natural products directly over a flame; instead, use a double boiler. Avoid trying to quickly cool products in the freezer or refrigerator. Best yet is to make fresh raw products!

Ingredients

Alcohol Rubbing alcohol (isopropyl alcohol) is an antiseptic, preservative, and solvent. When applied topically, it is cooling, cleansing, and astringent. It can also be drying. It has strong vapors that make some people feel sick. Never use isopropyl alcohol internally, even for things like mouthwashes. It is a petroleum by-product. Instead, use natural alcohols such as vodka, rum, or gin. Vodka is preferred because it is fragrance free. Heating alcohol can be a dangerous fire hazard.

Alfalfa (*Medicago sativa*) is a member of the Fabaceae (Pea) Family. The above-ground portion is used for its anti-inflammatory, moisturizing, nutritive, and tonic properties. Use as a tea internally to treat itchy skin. In cosmetics, it is included in facial steams for normal skin, as a soothing bath herb, and as a strengthening herb in hair rinses due to its high protein content. It is also included in poultices to treat wounds. Alfalfa is rich in chlorophyll, which promotes wound healing. It is naturally deodorizing and helps prevent infection.

Alkanet (*Alkanna tinctoria*) is a member of the Boraginaceae (Borage) Family. This beautiful blue flower has a root that yields a nontoxic natural red coloring when steeped in oil, ranging in hues from cherry to burgundy. It is used in making lip balms and blushers. It is astringent and antimicrobial and promotes wound healing.

Almonds (*Prunus dulcis*) are members of the Rosaceae (Rose) Family. When shelled, finely ground, and mixed with water, almonds can be used topically on skin for cleansing, smoothing, and softening. Almonds benefit dry skin as well as blackheads and enlarged pores. Almonds are excellent for removing dead and dry skin when used as a facial scrub or to exfoliate other rough areas, such as the elbows. When consumed, they are rich in protein, beta-carotene, and calcium, which nourishes the hair, skin, bones, and nails and calms troubled nerves.

Almond oil is good to use in aromatherapy products, as it is light, well absorbed, odorless, and improves the penetration of essential oils. It works well for normal and dry skin. Almond oil doesn't go rancid quickly, but it is best kept refrigerated once opened.

Aloe vera (*Aloe barbadensis*) is a member of the Liliaceae (Lily) Family. Known for the gelatinous substance in its stalks, aloe is appreciated for its cooling antibacterial, antifungal, anti-inflammatory, antiseptic, astringent, demulcent, emollient, preservative, moisturizing, rejuvenative, and vulnerary qualities. Aloe is reputed to have been one of the beauty secrets of Cleopatra. It is used topically to treat conditions such as acne, athlete's foot, boils, burns, dandruff, eczema, herpes, insect bites, poison ivy, poison oak, psoriasis, ringworm, scars, sunburn, wounds, and wrinkles. For people with acne, aloe vera can be taken internally: stir three ounces of aloe vera juice into a bit of water three times daily, and take about twenty minutes before each meal. Aloe vera is included in lotions, moisturizers, salves, soaps, sprays, toners, shampoos, and conditioners. If using fresh aloe, use the inner pulp, not the peel. Aloe vera products containing sorbic acid or potassium sorbate can cause a red and burning sensation in some people that lasts ten to fifteen minutes.

Alpha hydroxy acids are included in cosmetic products for their hydrating and exfoliating properties. The most common alpha hydroxy acids used in cosmetics include citric, glycolic, lactic, malic, and tartaric acids. Though glycolic acids do occur naturally in sugarcane, sugar beets, and unripe grapes, what is usually available commercially is synthetic.

Anise seeds (*Pimpinella anisum*) are members of the Apiaceae (Parsley) Family, with a lovely licorice-like scent. Anise is an anti-inflammatory agent and a mild stimulant. It is often included in facial steams to open the pores; it is also used as a facial cleanser and in hair rinses, soaps, and toner. It is used to flavor toothpastes and mouthwashes for its breath-freshening properties and is included in colognes. Both the herb and essential oil are used. As an essential oil, anise promotes relaxation and sleep and curbs sugar and chocolate cravings.

Annatto (*Bixa orellana*) is a member of the Bixaceae Family and native to the American tropics. The seeds are coated with a fleshy orange covering that yields a dye, which is why this plant is commonly referred to as "lipstick tree." It is one of the few natural dyes still used in the commercial cosmetic industry. It is also included as a coloring agent in rouges and hair rinses. Annatto is often found in herb stores and Hispanic markets.

Apple (*Malus species*) is a member of the Rosaceae (Rose) Family. Apples are antibacterial, anti-inflammatory, antiviral, astringent, and tonic. They improve skin diseases and facilitate weight loss. Eating apples stimulates saliva flow, promotes good digestion, cleans the teeth, prevents plaque buildup, and stimulates gum tissue. As a facial mask, puréed apples benefit dry, oily, and blemished skin and are mildly exfoliating. Apples are rich in flavonoids, beta-carotene, vitamins B and C, and the minerals boron, calcium, phosphorus, potassium, and silicon.

Apricots (*Prunus armeniaca*) are members of the Rosaceae (Rose) Family. They are laxative, due to their fiber and pectin content, nutritive, and considered alkaline and antioxidant. They have been used to treat acne. Apricots are rich in beta-carotene and vitamin C. Apricot pulp is used as a facial for tired, dry, or oily skin and to soften, prevent, and reduce the appearance of wrinkles. The seeds, when finely ground, are used topically for their exfoliating ability.

Arabic gum resin (*Acacia senegal*), also known as gum acacia, comes from a thorny African tree that is a member of the Fabaceae (Pea) Family. The resin is added to cosmetics as an emulsifier, binder, and stabilizer. It is considered safe enough to eat.

Arnica (*Arnica montana*) is a member of the Asteraceae (Daisy) Family. It is best and most often used as a homeopathic remedy or topically. Arnica is good to use for the aftermath of any trauma and to prevent postsurgical complications, such as swelling or pain, and to speed recovery. It is widely used for overexertion from athletic activities and painful muscles. A friend of mine, who is a plastic surgeon, suggests that his patients take homeopathic arnica before and after surgery to reduce the bruising that occurs from reconstruction. Arnica is often used as a compress, poultice, liniment, salve, or oil for back pain, bruises, chilblains, dislocations, phlebitis, rheumatic pain, sprains, and varicose veins. It should be used only on unbroken skin and not on exposed wounds. It speeds the healing process and helps restore normal sleep. Arnica has also been used topically to treat acne, couperose skin conditions, and varicosities. As a footbath, arnica comforts sore feet. Arnica is included in shampoos and conditioners as a hair growth stimulant to prevent hair loss and as a scalp tonic. It is believed that arnica increases the blood flow through affected capillaries, causing fluids that have escaped due to injury to be reabsorbed. Arnica aids in the resorption of fibrin, a blood protein resulting from internal injuries.

Arrowroot (*Maranta arundinacea*) is a member of the Marantaceae (Arrowroot) Family. The starch from the rhizome is demulcent and nutritive. It is used as a powder or bath herb (it may be added directly to bathwater) for heat rash and sunburn and to promote a smooth, silky feeling. In some countries arrowroot is used as a poultice for snakebites, insect bites, sores, and arrow wounds.

Avocado (*Persea americana*, *P. gratissima*) is a member of the Lauraceae (Laurel) Family. Avocado is rich in vitamins E and B complex, beta-carotene, potassium (it has two to three times more potassium than bananas), fluorine, copper, and lecithin. It is considered beautifying to the skin and hair when consumed. Those who have a difficult time digesting fats will usually find avocados easy to assimilate. An avocado has about 300 calories, and also contains the enzyme lipase, which aids in fat digestion. After enjoying this delectable fruit, rub the inside of the peel over your skin for a quick and effective moisturizer. Avocado can be used in facials and as a hair conditioner; simply mash the pulp, apply it to your face or scalp, and leave on for ten minutes before rinsing. It is especially good for dry and mature skin conditions. It soothes eczema and dry skin and scalp. Avocado oil is antioxidant and contains penetrating oils for very dry and mature skin. It is used for its sun protective and antioxidant properties.

Baking soda, also known as bicarbonate of soda, is used to clean almost everything. It is a gentle alkaline powder that neutralizes acids. It naturally dispels odors, lightens skin, and is anti-inflammatory. It helps absorb skin oils and exfoliates, tightens, and draws out toxins, leaving the skin smooth and soft. It is an excellent bath ingredient and helps relieve rashes and itchy skin. It also works as a water softener. Baking soda can be used for cleaning the teeth or as a facial scrub. It may be added to baths and to body powders. The powder is placed in shoes as a natural deodorizer.

Balsam of Peru (*Myroxylon balsamum*), a member of the Fabaceae (Pea) Family, is a tree that yields a vanilla-scented resin from its trunk. It is added to moisturizers and shampoos to impart moisture. Its essential oil is used as a perfume fixative.

Balsam of Tolu (*Myroxylon balsamum var. pereira*) is a close relative to balsam of Peru and is used in a similar fashion, yet it has a more subtle scent.

Bananas (*Musa paradisiaca*) are a member of the Musaceae (Banana) Family. Bananas are rich in carbohydrates, folic acid, vitamins C and B_6, potassium, and the fiber pectin. They provide long-term energy and improve stamina. They can improve sleep and elevate moods due to the presence of serotonin, a precursor to tryptophan and norepinephrine, which is needed for normal brain function. They are high in calories and can help people who are emaciated gain weight; bananas are a common food among Japanese sumo wrestlers. People on weight loss programs also use them, as they are low in fat and filling. Mashed bananas are applied as a facial to soothe and nourish sensitive, dry, normal, and fatigued skin and help the skin be free of impurities. The inner peel of a banana is sometimes used topically to treat warts, boils, frostbite, burns, and rashes.

Basil leaves (*Ocimum basilicum*) belong to the Lamiaceae (Mint) Family. The leaves are used for their antiseptic and circulatory-stimulating properties. Basil is used topically to treat acne, insect bites, and ringworm; it is also used as an insect repellent. The juice of the fresh plant is applied to fungal infections on the skin. Fresh and dried basil are included in salves and poultices. Basil is added to facial steams, cleansers, toners, and hair rinses, and its essential oil is used in soaps and perfumes. When added to hair products it imparts a delightful scent, improves hair growth, and tames tangles. Basil is made into a gargle or mouthwash for thrush, a bath herb for energy, and an eyewash for tired eyes. Both the herb and essential oil are used. Smelling basil essential oil can help us gain a second wind when we are fatigued. The essential oil is added to massage oils for sore muscles.

Bay (*Laurus nobilis*) is a member of the Lauraceae (Laurel) Family. Bay leaves are valued for their antifungal, antiseptic, and stimulating properties. They are used as a bath herb for sore muscles and joints. Bay leaf is included in facial steams. When used in shampoos, conditioners, and hair rinses, bay leaves help treat dandruff. Use bay leaf tea or seven drops of the essential oil diluted in a pan of warm water as a soak for nail fungus. The essential oil is used in perfumes and aftershaves and as an insect repellent. It is included in massage oil and liniments for sprains and arthritis. Bay leaves repel bugs and are thus included in potpourris and sachets.

Beer is rich in sugars and protein and excellent for adding volume to hair. Use it in a final rinse. Overuse will have a drying effect on the scalp and cause the hair to look dull.

Beeswax is the substance that bees use to make the walls of their honeycomb. It is naturally yellow with a delightful honey fragrance. White beeswax has been bleached by the sun and air. Beeswax is a natural emollient and a thickening and emulsifying agent that can make lotions and creams either hard or soft, depending on the amount of beeswax used. In general, about 1 ounce of beeswax is added to 2.5 ounces of oil to make a salve. There is a possibility of beeswax being allergenic to some people. Beeswax is not a vegan product, and for years I avoided bee products. However, we need bees to pollinate plants, and supporting small operations of ethical beekeepers that help protect the bees is important.

Bergamot (*Citrus bergamia*) is a member of the Rutaceae (Citrus) Family. It is antiseptic and sedative. The essential oil is inhaled to relieve anxiety, depression, and compulsive behavior, as well as to aid withdrawal from addiction to sugar, food, alcohol, cocaine, stimulants, or sedatives. In cosmetics, bergamot essential oil is used to help prevent scarring, though it can increase photosensitivity and should not be used before sun exposure.

Birch (*Betula alba*) is a member of the Betulaceae (Birch) Family. The leaf buds, leaves, inner bark, and sap are valued for their analgesic, antiseptic, astringent, and stimulant properties. Birch is incorporated into salves, washes, poultices, cleansers, and toners for acne, bruises, eczema, psoriasis, and wounds. It is an excellent bath herb for rashes and other skin eruptions. It is also used in facial steams in the treatment of acne. It is softening to the skin and included in shampoos, conditioners, and hair rinses to promote hair growth and to treat dandruff. It is included in toothpastes and toothache gel remedies for pain. Birch essential oil smells identical to wintergreen oil and is often substituted for the more expensive wintergreen.

Borax (sodium borate, also sodium tetraborate) is a naturally occurring white substance found on the alkaline shores of lakes in South America and the American Southwest. It is made of boron, sodium, oxygen, and water. It softens water and has a unique ability to suspend soap particles in water, making them less likely to clog pores or adhere to the skin, although some people find it irritates their skin. It is often added to bath salt products to prevent caking. Borax acts as a texturizer and binder, and when it is added to oil, water, and beeswax, it makes a stable emulsion. As a bath additive, it can help calm itchy skin.

Brazil nuts (*Bertholletia excelsa*) belong to the Lecythidaceae (Brazil Nut) Family. They are a good source of the amino acids cysteine and methionine, making them beneficial in a vegetarian diet and a good source of essential fatty acids. They are also a good source of selenium and are rich enough in calcium to be beneficial for teeth and bones. Brazil nut oil is rich in linoleic, alpha-linolenic, and palmitic acids. It is excellent in hair conditioners and will make the hair soft, silky, and bouncy. Rich in antioxidants, Brazil nut oil makes an excellent moisturizer. It is available as a raw food product.

Brewer's yeast (a by-product of the beer-making industry) and nutritional yeast (a delicious, primary-grown yeast) are nourishing and especially rich in B vitamins (some brands contain vitamin B_{12}) and protein. They are also deeply cleansing and tightening, and are good for oily skin and for enlivening dull-looking skin.

Burdock root (*Arctium lappa*) is a member of the Asteraceae (Daisy) Family. It is used internally and externally for skin conditions such as abscesses, acne, dandruff, eczema, hives, psoriasis, and ringworm. It improves lymphatic and liver health, and cleanses environmental and other toxins out of the system. Burdock aids in fat metabolism, and when used topically, it softens the skin. It is alterative, antifungal, anti-inflammatory, antiseptic, demulcent, diaphoretic, nutritive, and rejuvenative. The root is often added to facial steams, cleansers, lotions, toners, and salves; it is also used as a bath herb, especially for the treatment of oily and acne-prone skin. Burdock is added to shampoos, conditioners, and hair rinses, and is especially beneficial for dandruff and hair loss. Eat raw burdock as a vegetable, grated and added to salads.

Buriti oil (*Mauritia flexuosa*) is a member of the Palmaceae (Palm) Family. The edible nut is rich in beta-carotene. The juice can be consumed as a refreshing tonic. In Colombia it is made into a drink to strengthen the weak and elderly. The leaves are very emollient.

Calendula (*Calendula officinalis*) is a member of the Asteraceae (Daisy) Family. The beautiful yellow flowers are used for their antifungal, anti-inflammatory, antiseptic, astringent, demulcent, and vulnerary properties. When calendula is used either internally or externally, it helps increase peripheral circulation and improve skin conditions such as acne, boils, eczema, and psoriasis. A common ingredient in cosmetics, calendula is used in facial steams, cleansers, lotions, moisturizers, soaps, and salves. It helps refine pores and renews cells, and it is ideal for sensitive skin. An old saying is, "Where calendula is applied, no pus will form." Calendula soothes burns and sunburn. It is gentle enough to use in products such as eye creams and baby care products and can even help cradle cap and diaper rash. As a bath herb, calendula is used for dry skin. Calendula is used in shampoos, conditioners, and hair rinses, especially for blondes.

Camphor (*Cinnamomum camphora*) is a member of the Lauraceae (Laurel) Family. It is used in cosmetics for its antiseptic and antiacne properties.

Camu-camu fruit (*Myrciaria dubia*), a member of the Tamarix (Salt Cedar) Family, contains more vitamin C than any other known plant. It is also rich in calcium, iron, and niacin, and the amino acids leucine, serine, and valine. It is considered a powerful antioxidant. When consumed, camu-camu strengthens the immune system, lifts depression, improves energy, and helps relieve herpes and shingles. Simply add one-half teaspoon of powdered camu-camu in a glass of water three times daily to improve all the systems of the body. When added to hair products, such as shampoos and conditioners, it strengthens and imparts shine to the hair. It is considered nontoxic. Rain-forest dwellers are being encouraged to cultivate this plant to help the sustainability of the rain forest and its people.

Cantaloupe (*Cucumis melo*) is a member of the Cucurbitaceae (Gourd) Family. Melons are alkalinizing, antioxidant, cleansing, hydrating, laxative, and rejuvenative. They also function as a blood anticoagulant. Most melons are rich in fiber, pectin, vitamin C, flavonoids, vitamin B_6, potassium, carbohydrates, and protein. When the flesh is eaten close to the rind, they provide silicon. Melons are delightfully low in calories. They make the ideal food for breaking a fast, being one of the easiest foods to digest. People with diarrhea or who are feeling chilled should save melons for another time. As a facial mask, cantaloupe is pore tightening and refreshing; it may be used for both oily and dry skin.

Cardamom (*Elettaria cardamomum*) is a member of the Zingiberaceae (Ginger) Family. It is sweet, pungent, and warming, and when consumed, it is considered not only a digestive aid and breath freshener but an aphrodisiac. Its essential oil helps foster joy and is used in perfume, insect repellents, and massage oils.

Carnauba wax (*Copernicia cerifera*) is a natural product obtained from the wax exuded from the leaves of a Brazilian tree in the Palmaceae (Palm) Family. The tree protects itself during periods of drought by coating its leaves with a thick, waxy secretion. This waxy coating is collected, processed, and used in the manufacture of mascaras, lipsticks, and soaps.

Carrots (*Daucus carota sativa*) are members of the Apiaceae (Parsley) Family. Carrots have been used to treat acne, dry skin, eczema, and vision problems. Carrots are antibacterial, anti-inflammatory, antioxidant, astringent, and laxative. Eating a raw carrot daily exercises the teeth and jaw. Carrots are sweet, warm, and alkaline. Carrots contain beta-carotene, vitamins C and B_6, and calcium. Organic carrots can be eaten with the peel, which is beneficial for our skin. When blended into a purée and used as a facial mask, carrots help nourish the skin and treat blemishes, due to their antiseptic properties. Carrot masks are also good for dry skin.

Castor oil (*Ricinus communis*) is from the seed of a member of the Euphorbiaceae (Spurge) Family. It is included in lipsticks, lip balm, eyebrow pencils, creams, salves, lotions, soaps, and hairstyling products, as it moistens dry and mature skin, nourishes, and is deeply penetrating. It helps eliminate scars, heals cysts, and reduces eczema and psoriasis. It is included in bath oils for dry skin. The oil is obtained by macerating the crushed seed, without its coating, in alcohol. Any heat would extract the poison ricin. Compresses are usually made by saturating a clean piece of flannel with the oil. The compress is then applied to the body where needed, covered with a sheet of plastic, and warmed with a hot water bottle. Treatments are often done for ninety-minute periods: three days on, four days off, and then the procedure is resumed. Use only castor oil that is manufactured (not homemade), as ricin is extremely toxic. Clairvoyant Edgar Cayce called the castor bean plant "the palm of Christ."

Cedarwood (*Cedrus atlantica*) essential oil is antiseptic and antifungal and decreases oily secretions. The plant is a member of the Cedar Family. Cedar leaf oil, which is usually distilled from *Thuja occidentalis*, is used to treat warts.

Chamomile, German (*Matricaria recutita*) is a member of the Asteraceae (Daisy) Family. The flowers are used for their antibacterial, antifungal, anti-inflammatory, sedative, and vulnerary properties. Chamomile helps wound healing by promoting tissue granulation and epithelialization. Chamomile is often used in dry-skin formulas and to relax facial tension. It is added to cleansers, lotions, facial masks, soaps, salves, and eye creams; it is also used as a relaxing bath herb. It helps to cleanse the pores, clear acne, and reduce puffiness. Chamomile is excellent in salves and lotions for skin inflammations including burns, eczema, psoriasis, insect bites, and external ulcers, and to accelerate wound healing. Chamomile contains azulene, which brings out natural highlights when added to hair products. It is a favorite for blondes and is used in shampoos, conditioners, and hair rinses. Chamomile is used in massage oils for sore muscles and to promote relaxation. It is used as a gargle for sore throat and a mouthwash for gingivitis. Chamomile can be used as a poultice for toothaches and an eyewash for conjunctivitis and sties. It is even used as a douche and enema. Stuffed into a pillow, chamomile aids sleep. Its essential oil is added to calming massage blends and cooling spritzers. The essential oil can be used neat (undiluted) to the skin to calm irritation. Some people are allergic to chamomile and should avoid it.

Champa (*Michelia champaca*) essential oil yields a beautiful fragrance that is used in perfumery and in aromatherapy to dispel anger. It is also considered an aphrodisiac.

Chickweed (*Stellaria media*) is a member of the Caryophyllaceae (Pink) Family. The above-ground portion is esteemed for its alterative, anti-inflammatory, antiseptic, astringent, demulcent, diuretic, emollient, nutritive, pectoral, refrigerant, and vulnerary properties. Chickweed nourishes the *yin* fluids and is an herb traditionally given to strengthen the frail. Topical applications of chickweed include its use as a bath herb for dry skin and chicken pox, compress, poultice, and salve for boils, burns, diaper rash, hemorrhoids, eczema, itchy skin, nettle sting, psoriasis, and varicose veins. The fresh juice is applied to eyes in cases of infection, such as conjunctivitis. Allow fresh, wild chickweed to grow abundantly by your home and enjoy it in a daily green salad as often as possible.

Cinnamon bark (*Cinnamomum cassia. C. zeylanicum*) is a member of the Lauraceae (Laurel) Family. When used internally for a period of time, cinnamon helps to promote a rosy complexion. It is valued for its antifungal, antiseptic, aromatic, and astringent properties. Cinnamon is used in facial scrubs, soaps, cleansers, masks, and lotions. Its pungent sweet smell makes it desirable in perfumes and aftershaves. It is excellent for brunettes and to prevent baldness; it is included in shampoos and hair rinses for dark hair. When added to toothpastes and mouthwashes, it helps to freshen the breath. Cinnamon has been added to footbaths for athlete's foot. Used as a bath herb, it warms, chills, and relieves sore muscles. Considered an aphrodisiac, cinnamon essential oil is included in massage oils. The smell of cinnamon is pleasant and stimulates the senses, yet it calms the nerves. Its smell is reputed to attract customers to a place of business and cause them to linger longer, thus increasing prosperity.

Clary sage (*Salvia sclarea*) is a member of the Lamiaceae (Mint) Family. Its flowers and leaves are used for their aromatic and astringent properties. Clary sage is used for mature as well as acne-prone skin in cleansers, soaps, and toners. As a bath herb, clary sage helps relieve muscle tension and cramps as well as hormonal concerns related to premenstrual syndrome and menopause. For the hair, it is used in shampoos, conditioners, and hair rinses, and benefits dandruff and hair growth. The essential oil is included in perfumes, soaps, and powders. It is considered a relaxing agent and helps us feel more grounded in our bodies. Clary sage is an antidepressant, aphrodisiac, and mild euphoric.

Clay was used by the ancient Aztecs, Egyptians, and Mayans. Clay draws out toxins, clears the skin, improves circulation, and is cleansing and anti-inflammatory. Clay helps reduce large pores, firms sagging skin, and helps promote a clear and blemish-free complexion. Avoid using clay close to the eye area, as it can be too drying. Use only dry, cosmetic-quality clay. Do not use art clay for body care purposes; it has been processed and does not contain therapeutic properties. There are several types of high-quality, natural cosmetic clay available:

- Red clay is naturally high in iron and good for normal skin.
- Yellow clay is high in sulfur.
- Green clay is rich in calcium, chromium, copper, iron, magnesium, nickel, and silica. It is good for oily skin, as it reduces sebaceous secretions. Consider green clay to help clear up acne, eczema, hemorrhoids, psoriasis, and shingles.
- Blue clay is anti-inflammatory and useful for acne-prone, infected, and very sensitive skin. The blue color is due to the presence of natural cobalt.
- White clay is the mildest of all the cosmetic clays and is often included in body powders. White clay contains aluminum oxide, calcium, magnesium, silica, and zinc oxide. It balances sebaceous secretions and is recommended for all skin types, including dry and sensitive.
- Black and brown clays are rich in iron and zinc.
- Bentonite, found in Benton, Montana, is a fine gray clay, also known as fuller's earth. It is a volcanic ash and is rich in silica. Bentonite is used in facial masks to treat pimples and to dry up poison ivy. It is considered good for all skin types except sensitive.
- Kaolin clay is also known as China clay, as it was originally derived from Kaolin Hill in China. Both kaolin clay and bentonite are very useful for oily skin.

Cleavers (*Galium aparine*) is a member of the Rubiaceae (Madder) Family. The above-ground portion is primarily used internally as a tea, tincture, or in capsules to improve skin conditions such as acne, eczema, and psoriasis. It is an excellent lymphatic and kidney cleanser and is traditionally used in the springtime as a blood-purifying agent. It is used as a facial wash for acne, eczema, psoriasis, freckles, and loose, sagging skin. Topical applications of cleavers include a compress, poultice, or salve for burns, cancer, scars, eczema, poison ivy, psoriasis, sagging skin, stretch marks, sore nipples, spider bites, sunburn, and wounds.

Cloves (*Eugenia aromatica*) are a member of the Myrtaceae (Eucalyptus) Family. The dried flower buds are used for their antiseptic, aromatic, and astringent properties. Cloves are included in skin preparations such as soap, toner, lotion, perfume, powders, and aftershaves. Because cloves are antifungal, they are used in salves to treat athlete's foot. Cloves are used for brunettes and redheads in shampoos, conditioners, and hair rinses. They are used to flavor toothpastes and freshen the breath, and are used as a dental antiseptic, as cloves inhibit plaque formation. Suck on a clove for fresh breath. The essential oil is included in perfumes for its sensuous scent. It is applied on warts, insect bites (and is used as an insect repellent), and infected wounds. Clove is a popular scent in men's cosmetics. Clove essential oil is included in massage oils and liniments to ease neuralgia and rheumatism. It stimulates the thalamus in the brain to release enkephalin, a neurochemical that promotes a sense of euphoria and also gives pain relief.

Cocoa butter (*Theobroma cacao*) is a member of the Sterculiaceae Family. It is derived from the fat that surrounds the chocolate bean. Chocolate, made from the bean, is considered "food of the gods." The cocoa beans are pressed to yield the butter. Cocoa is a creamy, waxy, fatty substance that is solid at room temperature but melts at very low heat and when it comes in contact with the skin. It is used in lotions, creams, ointments, and soaps for dry skin, as it is very softening, emollient, and lubricating. It helps eliminate scars, is excellent for cracked dry skin and mature skin, and has some natural sun protective properties. It is also used as a natural thickening agent. Cocoa butter is very stable and not prone to going rancid. A bonus is that it smells like chocolate!

Coconut (*Cocos nucifera*), the largest known seed, is the fruit of the coconut palm tree, a member of the Palmaceae (Palm) Family. Coconuts are considered an energy tonic. They are 70 percent fat, most of which is saturated, but they can actually help the body break down fat and aid weight loss. Coconuts are high in iodine, which is important for normal thyroid function, and are a good source of protein, beta-carotene, B-complex vitamins, and minerals. They are excellent fare for vegetarians.

Coconut oil, also known as coconut butter, is solid at room temperature but becomes a clear liquid at temperatures greater than 78 degrees F. In the body, it is quickly burned for energy production. Coconut oil smells great and imparts beauty and radiance when rubbed on the skin. It is excellent for inflamed and sensitive skin as well as normal, dry, mature, and oily skin. It blocks about 20 percent of UV rays. Coconut oil is used in massage oils, skin care products, and first aid creams to heal tissue and prevent scarring. People who suffer from psoriasis may benefit from topical applications of coconut oil. It is very nourishing, cooling, and moisturizing and has a long shelf life. It adds shine to hair and is used as a hot oil and scalp treatment to impart strength and glossiness to the hair. Be sure to use only cold-pressed or expeller pressed oils to avoid harmful trans fats.

Comfrey (*Symphytum officinale*) is a member of the Boraginaceae (Borage) Family. The leaves and flowers are used topically for their anti-inflammatory, emollient, and regenerative properties. Comfrey contains allantoin, which stimulates new cell growth. Comfrey is excellent for dry skin and wrinkled skin. It is included in soaps, lotions, moisturizers, and salves, and is used as a bath herb to soothe, smooth, and deter aging of the skin. Comfrey is included in lotions, poultices, and salves to treat bruises, burns, eczema, hemorrhoids, scars, swellings, wounds, wrinkles, sunburn, and varicosities. Excellent for dry hair and dandruff, comfrey is used in shampoos, conditioners, and hair rinses. Comfrey is not suggested for internal use, unless recommended by a qualified health practitioner.

Coriander (*Coriandrum sativum*) is a member of the Apiaceae (Parsley) Family. The seeds are used for their antifungal, aromatic, and stimulating qualities. Coriander is used in lotions and as a bath herb for sore muscles and joints. The essential oil is used to flavor toothpastes, as it is breath freshening. Its pleasant fragrance in valued in perfumery, aftershaves, and soaps. The essential oil is motivating, a gentle stimulant, and helps relieve depression and stress. It has long been used in love potions and as an aphrodisiac.

Cornflower (*Centaurea sativum*, *C. cyanus*) is a member of the Asteraceae (Daisy) Family. It is also known as "bachelor's button." It is a gentle astringent and useful as a facial spray, facial steam, toner, eye cream, and compress for puffy eyes. It is also used in antiwrinkle creams and lotions. Cornflower is included in hair rinses for blonde, gray, and white hair.

Cornmeal is made from ground corn (*Zea mays*), a member of the Poaceae (Grass) Family. It is included in facial scrubs as an exfoliating agent.

Corn silk is the silky threads from fresh ears of corn. They can be dried in a warm room in a paper bag. When finely ground, they make a silky powder.

Cornstarch is used in powders to soothe the skin. Be aware that much corn grown in the United States is genetically modified, and we don't fully know how that might affect human health.

Cotton balls (*Gossypium hirsutum*, *G. herbaceum*) are made from cotton, a member of the Malvaceae (Malva) Family. Use real cotton, as cosmetic "puffs" can be made of irritating ingredients that come off on your skin. Since cotton is one of the most highly sprayed crops on the planet, organic cotton is best for your skin and the planet.

Cucumber (*Cucumis sativus*) is a member of the Cucurbitaceae (Gourd) Family. It has a high silicon content (especially in the peel) that encourages healthy skin, nails, and hair growth. Cucumbers are considered therapeutic for those suffering from acne, obesity, and sunburn. Mashed cucumber is applied topically to cool burns, wasp stings, and tired, swollen feet. Cooling, astringent, and soothing, cucumber is used in lotions, facials, and compresses for acne, oily skin, sensitive skin, enlarged pores, freckles, sunburn, and wrinkles. It helps reduce puffiness and inflammation. Cucumber slices can be applied to puffy, tired eyes to reduce redness and inflammation. Commercial cucumbers often have wax on their skins, which should not be eaten.

Cypress (*Cupressus sempervirens*) is a member of the Cupressaceae (Cypress) Family. The essential oil is used in cosmetics for its antiseptic, astringent, sedative, and styptic properties. It is a specific ingredient in anti-cellulite lotions and massage oils.

Dandelion (*Taraxacum officinale*) is a member of the Asteraceae (Daisy) Family. Drinking a tea of dandelion root is one of the best skin treatments to ensure beauty from the inside out, as it helps purify the blood by improving liver function. Dandelion root tea is a supreme internal remedy for acne, boils, eczema, psoriasis, and sallow skin. The leaves, blossoms, and roots are nutritive and antifungal. They are included in facial steams and masks and are used as a wash or compress for acne, eczema, psoriasis, and wounds. Adding dandelion to the bath helps remedy eczema and dry, oily, or itchy skin. Dandelion is also used to promote weight loss. The sap from the stem can be applied to warts to make them disappear. Learn to eat young dandelion greens in salads as a true beauty food!

Echinacea (*Echinacea purpurea*, *E. angustifolia*) is a member of the Asteraceae (Daisy) Family. The root, leaves, flowers, and seeds are used internally for their antifungal, anti-inflammatory, antiseptic, and vulnerary properties to remedy skin conditions such as abscesses, acne, boils, and eczema. Echinacea stimulates white blood cell and interferon production, and makes cells less susceptible to viral takeover. It can also help regenerate cells that have been damaged. Topically, echinacea is used in compresses, salves, and poultices to treat infected wounds and insect bites. Apply the tincture directly to a pimple to help dry it up quickly.

Eclipta (*Eclipta alba*) is a member of the Asteraceae (Daisy) Family. The entire plant is made into an oil and used topically on the scalp to curb hair loss and graying and to promote luster. It is considered anti-inflammatory, rejuvenative, and tonic. Drinking a tea of eclipta promotes beautiful skin.

Elder (*Sambucus nigra*, *S. canadensis*) is a member of the Caprifoliaceae (Honeysuckle) Family. The flowers are used for their anti-inflammatory, emollient, and mild astringent properties. Elder blossoms are used for acne, oily, dry, and wrinkled skin in facial steams, cleansers, scrubs, lotions, moisturizers, soaps, toners, and salves. It is reputed to help clean clogged pores. Elder flower water is a classic toner, reputed to be one of the beauty secrets of many women of the seventeenth century. It makes a good aftershave and has been used to lighten freckles and skin discolorations, calm sunburn, and reduce enlarged pores and eye puffiness when used as a compress. Elder flowers make a relaxing bath herb. Elder benefits dry hair when used in shampoos, conditioners, and hair rinses. When used internally as a tea or tincture, elder helps to clean the pores from the inside. Elderberry juice has also been used to color lips and cheeks. Elderberries have traditionally been used to darken graying hair.

Epsom salts (magnesium sulfate) are originally from Epsom, England. These colorless or white crystals have anti-inflammatory and muscle-relaxing effects and are often added to the bath and to make bath salts. During World War I, Epsom salt baths were used to treat shell shock. Daily use can be drying.

Eucalyptus (*Eucalyptus globulus*) is a member of the Myrataceae (Eucalyptus) Family. The leaves and twigs are appreciated for their antiseptic, aromatic, astringent, and mildly stimulating properties. Eucalyptus is used in deodorants, salves, and soaps. Eucalyptus helps decongest clogged sinuses and is included in facial steams, chest rubs, and massage oils and liniments for sore muscles. It makes an excellent invigorating bath herb for muscle and joint soreness, sunburn, and respiratory congestion. Eucalyptus is included in shampoos, conditioners, and hair rinses to treat dandruff. The tea can be used as a gargle for throat infections and as a breath-freshening mouthwash. It makes an antiseptic and deodorant footbath. Eucalyptus yields one of the most antiseptic of the essential oils, which is diluted and used topically for blisters, boils, burns, herpes, sores, and wounds. It is made into salves, deodorants, insect repellents, and massage oil, and is used for decongesting the chest and sinuses, headaches, painful arthritic joints, athletic recovery, and stiff joints. The oil is used in steam baths, saunas, and vapor inhalations. It can be inhaled as a decongestant and to prevent fainting.

Fennel (*Foeniculum vulgare*) is a member of the Apiaceae (Parsley) Family. The fennel seed and bulb are traditionally used in the Mediterranean to curb appetite and promote slenderness, as they naturally stabilize blood sugar levels. The seeds are used for their anti-inflammatory and aromatic properties for mature skin in facial steams, cleansers, soaps, antiwrinkle creams, and lotions. It helps to calm unevenly colored, blotchy skin. A cool fennel-seed-tea compress is used to reduce puffiness on closed, swollen eyes. It is included in salves to heal bruises. Chewing a few fennel seeds after a meal helps to freshen the breath. The essential oil is used in perfume, to scent shampoos, and to flavor toothpastes and mouthwashes. Folklore recommends fennel for promoting courage, self-esteem, and strength. Considered a tonic for the female reproductive system due to its phytoestrogenic activity, fennel is often included in breast-enlargement capsules.

Frankincense (*Boswellia carterii*) is a member of the Burseraceae (Frankincense) Family. The resin of this plant has a long tradition of being used for its analgesic, anti-inflammatory, aromatic, antiseptic, immune stimulating, and rejuvenative properties. It is used in facial steams and cleansers and toners for mature skin, acne, boils, scars, and varicose veins. It is used as a salve or liniment to treat rheumatism, wounds, and sports injuries. It is included in mouthwashes as an antiseptic agent. Long used in perfumery, frankincense is still burned as incense, including in hospitals to prevent the spread of infectious diseases. Its essential oil is used in antiaging formulas and in preparations to prevent skin cancer.

Geranium (*Geranium* and *Pelargonium species*) is a member of the Geraniaceae (Geranium) Family. The roots and leaves are powerful astringents and anti-inflammatory agents. Geranium is used in facial steams, toners, masks, antiwrinkle creams, and soaps for mature and oily skin. Geranium is also used for oily hair in shampoos, conditioners, and rinses. Scented geraniums, under the genus of *Pelargonium*, are included in facial steams, bath mixtures, hair rinses, perfumes, and soaps for their aromatic and rejuvenative properties. The essential oil is used to calm anxiety, reduce stress and fatigue, and stimulate sensuality. Geranium helps us feel at ease, improves relationships, and aids in resolving passive-aggressive tendencies. It is a thyroid stimulant, antidepressant, antiseptic, aphrodisiac, cell regenerator, and hormonal balancer for men and women.

Gingerroot (*Zingiber officinale*) is a Zingiberaceae (Ginger) Family member. Hawaiian ginger, which is popular in hair products, is called *awapuhi*. Ginger rhizomes are used as an antibacterial, antifungal, anti-inflammatory, antioxidant, antiseptic, aromatic, and circulatory stimulant. Ginger compresses are applied on arthritic joints, bunions, and sore muscles. Ginger is used as a bath herb for chills, muscle soreness, sciatica, and poor circulation. It is used in foot soaks, massage oils, and as a bath herb for athlete's foot, colds, and flu. A Chinese folk remedy is to rub the cut root on the scalp to stop hair loss and dandruff. The essential oil is used in men's aftershaves. Ginger is included in perfumes, sachets, and potpourris for its spicy fragrance. Its stimulating aroma helps open the heart and is aphrodisiac, even benefiting erectile dysfunction. It improves circulation and depression.

Ginseng, American (*Panax quinquefolius*) and **Ginseng, Asian** (*Panax ginseng*) are members of the Araliaceae (Ivy) Family. The Chinese say that ginseng helps crystallize the earth's energy and benefits that energy the body has lost. Ginseng has one of the longest recorded histories of use, going back some 6,000 years. It has been valued for its restorative properties and as an energy tonic. Ginseng root (both varieties) is used as an adaptogen, anti-inflammatory, antioxidant, nutritive, rejuvenative, restorative, stimulant, and tonic. Ginseng is included in antiwrinkle facial products, as it helps heal, nourish, and soften the skin.

Glycerin is a triatomic alcohol (glycerol) by-product that can be derived from alcohol, animal fats, or distilled from vegetable oils. Synthetic glycerin is derived from propylene glycol, a petrochemical that can be irritating to the skin and scalp. Propylene glycol is added to cosmetic products as an emulsifier, to keep products from separating. It can clog pores and cause allergic reactions. I recommend using only pure vegetable glycerin. A colorless, sticky syrup, glycerin is antiseptic, emollient, humectant, and lubricating. Pure natural glycerin has been used for hundreds of years to lubricate the skin (as with rose water and glycerin) and to preserve and dilute cosmetics. When there is a high degree of humidity in the atmosphere, glycerin helps carry moisture to the skin. Glycerin preserves the skin's natural protection by filling in the intercellular matrix and attracting enough water to maintain the skin's homeostasis. However, there are some experts who argue that glycerin drains the skin of moisture and can be irritating to sensitive skin, even causing it to become moisture depleted in the long run.

Goldenseal (*Hydrastis canadensis*) is a member of the Ranunculaceae (Crowfoot) Family. The root is used internally for its antiseptic properties to treat acne, boils, impetigo, and skin infections. Topically, it is used in washes, compresses, poultices, and salves to treat conditions such as athlete's foot, eczema, herpes, impetigo, poison ivy, ringworm, and wounds. It makes an excellent gargle for mouth sores, sore throat, thrush, pyorrhea, and gum infections, and powdered goldenseal is used for tooth and gum infections. Goldenseal has been overharvested from the wild, and although it is a very valuable herb, we need to cultivate it and bring this plant back to thriving levels before it should be taken from its natural habitat. Pregnant women and people with very low blood sugar levels should avoid internal use of goldenseal. Long-term use can kill off friendly intestinal flora.

Gotu kola (*Centella asiatica*) is a member of the Apiaceae (Parsley) Family. The above-ground portions are used for their rejuvenative properties. Gotu kola helps strengthen connective tissue, enhances collagen production, improves circulation, softens the skin, promotes wound and scar healing by stimulating cellular mitosis, and promotes tensile integrity of the tissue. It is taken internally in the form of tea, tincture, or capsules to treat age spots, burns, cellulite, dermatitis, eczema, leprosy, psoriasis, and scars (even the keloid variety). Gotu kola is included in baths, salves, lotions, and moisturizers to help burns, eczema, and psoriasis.

Grapefruit seed extract (*Citrus paradisi*), sometimes referred to as citracidal, is a member of the Rutaceae (Citrus) Family. It is used as a preservative in some cosmetics. Grapefruit seed extract is an antibacterial, antifungal, and antioxidant. It is used to treat many bugaboos such as *Aspergillus*, *Candida*, *Chlamydia*, cholera, diarrhea, *E. coli*, *Entamoeba histolytica*, flu, *Giardia*, herpes, parasites, pseudomonas, *Salmonella*, *Shigella*, *Staphylococcus*, *Streptococcus* (the cause of strep throat), and *Trichophyton*. It is available as a liquid extract or in capsules. Follow the directions according to the manufacturer's suggestions. Grapefruit seed extract is included in mouthwashes and gargles for gum infection, halitosis, and sore throat. Diluted, it is used in ears for ear infections, as a nasal rinse for sinus infections, as a douche for yeast infections, and as a facial cleanser for acne. Apply grapefruit seed extract to warts, athlete's foot, and nail fungus, and use it as a wash for poison oak. It can also be used in a hair rinse for dandruff. This substance is very refined, and sometimes it is more synthetic than natural; however, it has many valuable applications for the herbal practitioner. Always dilute the liquid extract, as it can be caustic, and do not get it into your eyes. Rinse with cool water for ten minutes if direct contact with mucous membranes occurs.

Grapes (*Vitis vinifera*) are members of the Vitaceae (Grape) Family. Grapes contain beta-carotene, B-complex vitamins, and vitamin C. They are antibacterial, antiviral, and diuretic. Grape skins contain resveratrol, which prevents blood platelet aggregation and elevates the beneficial HDL cholesterol. The darker varieties (red and purple) are more beneficial than the white or green varieties and are considered better for building blood, as they are richer in iron; they also contain the antioxidant quercetin. Grapes with their seeds intact are rich in antioxidant flavonoids, which are used to treat varicose veins. Grapes can be used in facials to cleanse, cool, lighten, and tighten all types of skin.

Grapeseed oil is light and astringent and a good carrier oil for aromatherapy. It is excellent for normal to oily skin.

Guggulu (*Commiphora mukul*) is a member of the Burseraceae (Frankincense) Family. The resin is used as a rejuvenative, stimulant, and thyroid tonic. Guggulu contains phytosterols and helps lower harmful low-density lipoprotein while elevating the beneficial high-density lipoprotein. It helps prevent blood platelet aggregation and breaks up already formed blood clots. Because it helps activate thyroid function by improving iodine assimilation, it may encourage weight loss. It stimulates circulation, promotes flexibility, and increases energy. Guggulu promotes bowel regularity as well as the secretion of digestive juices.

Gum benzoin (*Styrax benzoin*) is a member of the Styraceae Family. This yellow-beige fragrant resin of a tropical tree acts as a perfume fixative, antibacterial agent, and astringent. It also works as an emulsifier and preservative. Gum benzoin is included in creams, soaps, and lotions, as it prevents fats from becoming rancid. Its synthetic version, sodium benzoate, is found more commonly.

Gymnema (*Gymnema sylvestre*), also known as "gurmar," is a member of the Asclepiadaceae (Milkweed) Family. Gymnema has long been used to treat obesity. Gurmar means "sugar destroyer," and when people chew some of this leaf and then place sugar on their tongue, the sweet taste is eliminated in a few seconds. The molecules of the gymnemic acid fill the receptor sites for one to two hours, thus preventing the taste buds from being activated by the sugar molecules in food; it actually blocks sugar from being absorbed during digestion. It improves glucose utilization, enhances insulin production, and helps one overcome sugar addiction. It contains stigmasterol, betaine, and choline. If you are using gymnema and are insulin dependent, consult with your physician, as your insulin medication may need to be adjusted.

Hawthorn (*Crataegus species*) is a member of the Rosaceae (Rose) Family. Hawthorn leaves, flowers, and berries are used as a circulatory stimulant, diuretic, nervine, nutritive, and rejuvenative. It is used to treat obesity and calms the spirit. In Asian medicine, hawthorn is used more as a digestive aid, whereas in Western medicine, it is considered more of a heart tonic. Hawthorn can be used to strengthen joint lining, collagen, and discs in the back and to help one better retain a chiropractic adjustment. Hawthorn is effective as a medicine for softening hard substances and aids in the digestion of fats and oils. Hawthorn contains vitamin C, choline, acetylcholine, vitamins B_1 and B_2, calcium, tartaric acid, and flavonoids. Using hawthorn may increase the effects of heart medications such as beta-blockers. Consult with a competent health professional, as the medication dosage may need to be lowered. It is considered extremely safe.

Hazelnuts (*Corylus avellana*) are members of the Corylaceae (Hazel) Family. The wild nut is known as a hazelnut; the cultivated nut is called a filbert. Both strengthen teeth and gums, are acid forming, and are rich in calcium and other minerals. Hazelnut oil, which is light and rich, is sometimes added to formulas for oily skin. It is also used as a sun-protective oil.

Hempseed (*Cannabis sativa*) belongs to the Cannabaceae (Hemp) Family. Recent tests in Germany indicate that hempseed oil, when used in creams and lotions, is less sticky and penetrates the skin better than products made with other vegetable oils. Hempseed oil has a wide variety of cosmetic uses in salves, baby creams, soaps, shower gels, massage oils, lip balms, and lipsticks. Hempseed oil can replenish the oils of dry skin and help promote rapid healing of irritated tissues, bringing a youthful vitality to the skin. For hair care, hempseed oil is used in shampoos to relieve dry, itchy scalp. In Asian countries, hempseed oil is applied topically to the scalp to prevent hair loss. The lipids of hempseed enhance shine, improve manageability, and add body to hair. The ancient Chinese medical text the *Pen T'sao* says, "If one's head is washed with this, the hair will accelerate its growth and be properly balanced with just the right amount of moisture." Thus far, no allergic reactions have been reported by consumers from using hempseed oil topically. Using hempseed oil in cosmetics will not cause any psychoactive effects or cause you to have a positive drug test. For more information on hemp, check out *The HempNut Cookbook* by Richard Rose, Brigitte Mars, and Christina Pirello (Book Publishing Company, 2004). This is truly a plant that can help heal people and our planet!

Henna (*Lawsonia alba*, *L. inermis*) is a member of the Lythraceae (Henna) Family. The flowers and leaves from this Middle Eastern and African shrub make a delicate perfume and facial wash. The leaves are popular as a hair colorant and have also been used to make temporary tattoos, decorating the palms of the hands, soles of the feet, and fingernails with a reddish tint. As a hair coloring, henna coats the hair shaft and adds body and shine without penetrating it. It is used in shampoos, conditioners, and hair rinses. Henna can be used on all types of hair, but it is especially beneficial for oily hair. It helps loosen scalp buildup and prevents flaking and irritation. When using henna, avoid metal utensils (especially aluminum), which can react with the henna and cause the color to change. Also, be sure to buy pure henna that does not contain metallic salts, as these can create a toxic buildup in the hair. Some henna has had its coloring agent, lawsone, removed, so that the henna is used as a conditioning agent without changing the hair's color. Avoid using henna if you already color or perm your hair, as you may get some surprising effects, such as green hair.

Hibiscus (*Hibiscus rosa-sinensis*) is a member of the Malvaceae (Malva) Family. The leaves and flowers are valued for their emollient properties. They are included in facial steams for dry skin. The flowers impart a reddish tint to the hair when used as a rinse. The leaves yield a mucilage that can be used as a shampoo for dry hair. Asian women mix hibiscus flowers with oil to stimulate hair growth and treat dandruff. In China, the juice of the petals is used to darken the eyebrows. Hibiscus blossoms are edible and add beauty to any dish. Share one with your beloved.

Honey is mildly antiseptic and emollient and moisturizing. It helps draw impurities out of the skin and is favored for both dry and oily skin. It helps soothe, heal, and nourish the skin. It is good for lackluster skin, enlarged pores, and blackheads. Try applying honey on your face and neck then gently tapping over the area for two minutes. Rinse well. Add a teaspoon of honey to shampoo to condition your hair as you wash it. Use only raw honey that is righteously shared with the bees.

Honeysuckle (*Lonicera japonica*) is a member of the Caprifoliaceae (Honeysuckle) Family. Its flowers are used in cosmetics for their antifungal, antiseptic, astringent, and refrigerant qualities. It is included in lotions and moisturizers for its skin-softening and antiwrinkle treatment properties. Honeysuckle is used in washes and compresses to treat bruises, poison oak and ivy, rashes, sunburn, and swellings.

Hoodia (*Hoodia gordonii*) looks like a cactus but it's actually a succulent in the Asclepiadaceae (Milkweed) Family from the Kalahari Desert in southern Africa. Bushmen from the area have been using hoodia for centuries to help ward off hunger during long trips in the desert. Hoodia tricks the brain into thinking you've eaten and makes you feel full. Studies show that it reduces interest in food, delays the time after eating before hunger sets in again, and promotes a full feeling more quickly. It contains a substance known as P57 that is believed to suppress the appetite by affecting the nerve cells that send the brain glucose, causing one to feel satisfied. It is not a stimulant and has no known side effects.

Horse chestnut (*Aesculus hippocastanum*) is a member of the Hippocastanaceae (Horse Chestnut) Family. The seeds and bark are valued for their astringent and circulatory stimulant properties. They are used internally and topically to strengthen fragile capillaries and reduce cellulite, eczema, and varicose veins. They are high in flavonoids and a compound called aescin, which is anti-inflammatory.

Horsetail (*Equisetum arvense*) is a member of the Equisetaceae (Horsetail) Family. The above-ground portion is used cosmetically for its nutritive ingredients, especially silica and sulfur. Regularly drinking horsetail tea helps to strengthen hair, bones, and nails and prevent their brittleness. Horsetail is used in facial steams, toners, and lotions; it is excellent for oily skin and enlarged pores. It is used in shampoos, conditioners, and hair rinses for oily hair and dandruff; it also strengthens fragile hair. It is included in nail soaks as a strengthener. Horsetail is used as a poultice for wounds to stop bleeding and promote healing. It is made into a foot soak for malodorous and sweaty feet. As a mouthwash, it helps gingivitis and canker sores. As a compress, it treats eye inflammation and conjunctivitis. It is used as a bath herb for poor circulation and weak skin tone.

Irish moss (*Chrondus crispus*) is a member of the Gigartinaceae Family. It has anti-inflammatory, demulcent, and emollient properties and is highly nutritive. It is included in lotions and moisturizers to soften and moisturize dry skin and prevent wrinkles. A compress or poultice is applied to inflamed tissues. It is also used to thicken cosmetics, such as toothpaste.

Jasmine (*Jasminum species*) is a member of the Oleaceae (Olive) Family. The flowers provide one of the most delightful fragrances on earth and are considered an aphrodisiac. They are included in facial sprays, bath herbs, lotions, massage oil, and eye creams to benefit dry, mature, and sensitive skin. The dried or fresh flowers make a relaxing bath herb. Jasmine flowers are used as a compress for tired and inflamed eyes. Jasmine essential oil is used in perfume and soap and to scent shampoos, conditioners, and hair rinses. Every week, wash your hairbrush and then apply two to three drops of jasmine essential oil to the bristles for beautifully scented hair that is a pleasure to brush. If you live where jasmine grows, weave some flowers into your hair for beauty and fragrance. Many consider the aroma of jasmine to foster feelings of love, confidence, compassion, receptivity, and physical and emotional well-being. The essential oil has a chemical structure similar to human sweat and helps stimulate dopamine production. It is easily absorbed and mixes with human pheromones. It is believed to increase the attractiveness of whoever wears it. It also relieves stress, helps move emotional blocks, calms fear, alleviates anxiety, and is mildly euphoric. The pure essential oil is very expensive. If you pay a cheap price for it, expect that it has been adulterated. It is available more often as an absolute, which is not a pure essential oil. Jasmine is sacred to Kama, the Hindu god of love (an Eastern version of Cupid), who had jasmine on the tip of one of his arrows.

Jojoba oil (*Simmondsia chinensis*) is from a desert shrub that can survive hundreds of years at temperatures as high as 122 degrees F. It was used for centuries by the Apache Indians and Indians of Mexico as a scalp tonic. Jojoba is technically a liquid wax that is often compared to the whale by-product spermaceti, which also means that its use can help decrease whale hunting. As it closely resembles sebum of the scalp, it helps dissolve embedded sebum and is ideal for hair products. It helps prevent an oily scalp and hair loss due to clogged pores. Jojoba is good for oily, acne-prone, dry, damaged, and mature skin and doesn't feel oily on the skin. It has a long, stable shelf life and does not turn rancid, even when not refrigerated.

Juniper (*Juniperus communis*) is a member of the Cupressaceae (Cypress) Family. The berries (which are ripe when they turn blue) are antifungal, anti-inflammatory, and antiseptic. The essential oil of juniper is added to massage oil or used as a bath herb for sore joints, muscles, rheumatism, and cellulite. It is used in salves for acne, eczema, and psoriasis, and added to hair rinses for dandruff and alopecia. To this day, juniper is still burned in temples for purification and in villages during epidemics. It repels insects.

Kelp (*Fucus versiculosus*) is a member of the Fucaceae Family. The entire plant is valued for its detoxifying, mucilaginous, and nutritive properties. Using kelp internally in tablets or as an addition to food nourishes the bones, hair, and nails. Being rich in iodine, it nourishes the thyroid gland. By activating the thyroid gland and improving metabolism, kelp helps reduce cellulite and aids weight loss. Kelp is added to slimming soaps, baths, and thigh creams. Kelp is used in masks, toners, and lotions for its antiaging properties. It helps to soften and revitalize the skin. For oily hair and to promote shine, kelp is included in shampoos, conditioners, and hair rinses. Learn to love and eat sea vegetables regularly.

Khella (*Ammi visnaga*) is a member of the Apiaceae (Parsley) Family. It is antiallergenic, aromatic, and vasodilating. The fruit is used internally and also in salves topically to treat vitiligo. Khella, which contains the compound khellin, helps to stimulate the synthesis of the skin pigment melanin.

Kokum butter (*Garcinia indica*), also known as Goa butter, is a solid white fat from the fruit of the kokum palm. It helps promote skin elasticity and reduces degeneration. It is included in lotions, soaps, and salves for its emollient properties. Do not use kokum butter raw.

Kukui nut (*Aleurites moluccana*) is a member of the Euphorbiaceae (Spurge) Family. Native to Hawaii, it is also known as candlenut tree. Kukui nut is high in essential fatty acids and easily absorbed by the skin. It is helpful in lotions for dry skin, acne, eczema, and sunburn. It is an excellent addition to lip balms and is very emollient. The nuts have been used as torches by stringing them on the midrib of a coconut leaf.

Lady's-mantle (*Alchemilla vulgaris*) is a member of the Rosaceae (Rose) Family. The genus name *Alchemilla* is from the Arabic *alkemelych*, meaning "alchemy," as alchemists believed that the morning crystal dewdrops in this plant, which they called "heaven's water," held magical powers to help them in their work.

The common name "lady's-mantle" is in reference to a woman's cloak, presumably the Virgin Mary's, though in earlier times it was an herb of the goddess Freya. The leaves and flowering shoots are used as an anti-inflammatory, astringent, styptic agent, tonic, and vulnerary. Lady's-mantle is bitter, warm, and dry. Lady's-mantle promotes tissue healing and calms the spirit. It strengthens muscles and tissues and helps restore vitality after childbirth. A compress is applied to the skin and breasts to keep them firm and young-looking, especially after breast-feeding. Topically, lady's-mantle is used as a poultice for wounds. It is used as an eyewash for conjunctivitis, a mouthwash for sores and after dental extractions, and a gargle for laryngitis. The juice and tea are applied to acne. The tea is used as a facial steam for acne. Lady's-mantle is included in lotions to soften rough skin, lighten freckles, and minimize enlarged pores, wrinkles, and birthmarks. It has long been used as a method to stop excessive bleeding.

Lavender (*Lavandula species*) is a member of the Lamiaceae (Mint) Family. The word "lavender" is actually derived from the Latin *lavare*, meaning "to wash," as this herb has such a long tradition in cleansing. The flowers are highly aromatic, antiseptic, and astringent. Lavender is used in skin formulas including facial steams, cleansers, toners, lotions, and soaps to treat conditions such as acne, eczema, and psoriasis; it benefits all types of skin. Lavender is included in shampoos, conditioners, and hair rinses to impart a beautiful fragrance. It is an excellent bath herb that helps to lift the spirits after a difficult day. Lavender regenerates cells and helps to prevent wrinkles and scarring when the essential oil is added to lotions and salves. Lavender essential oil is applied to burns and sunburns and is one of the only essential oils that can be applied undiluted to the skin. A drop or two of undiluted lavender essential oil is applied topically to dispel a pimple that wants to erupt. Misting yourself several times daily with lavender water helps to moisturize the skin and will improve your mood. A foot soak in lavender tea or water scented with the essential oil is great for tired, achy feet. Lavender oil is included in massage oils for its ability to uplift the emotions and soothe muscles. Lavender is an important perfume ingredient. Place a few drops of lavender oil on your hairbrush after washing your brush to impart fragrance and stimulate hair growth. Long live lavender!

Lemon (*Citrus limon*) is a member of the Rutaceae (Citrus) Family. Lemons are sour, cooling, alkaline, antiseptic, and astringent. They contain citric acid, which exfoliates and encourages the growth of healthy cells. Lemon is used in skin care products for lightening uneven pigment, liver spots, and even scars. Lemon juice can be applied topically to calm itchy insect bites, pimples, corns, warts, boils, and poison ivy. Lemon juice helps to tighten enlarged pores, but it should be diluted with water before using. Lemon is added to hair rinses as a highlighter, to refresh the scalp, and to promote shiny hair. It can also be used as a hair spray, hand cleanser, and to restore the skin's acid mantle. Consume lemons for liver health, bone health, to strengthen connective tissues, and to repair damaged cells. Due to their high acidity, sucking on lemons can damage dental enamel. Avoid spending time in the sun after applying lemon to your skin, as it can cause photosensitivity. Lemon essential oil is antidepressant and emotionally cleansing. It helps relieve irritability and insomnia. Lemon is antiseptic, antifungal, and lithotropic.

Lime (*Citrus aurantifolia*) has the same properties and uses as lemon.

Lemon balm (*Melissa officinalis*) is a member of the Lamiaceae (Mint) Family. It was included in Carmelite Water, a popular toilet water used by men and women in medieval Europe. The leaves are used in facial steams and toners for blemishes and as a rejuvenative agent. Topically, lemon balm is used as a compress or poultice for swellings such as boils, burns, eczema, gout, headache, insect bites, shingles, sunburn, and tumors. It makes a comforting bath herb and is good for improving stress and a bad mood. Lemon balm is also included in shampoos, conditioners, and hair rinses for its lovely lemon scent and its ability to stimulate hair growth. The essential oil is diluted and used topically on herpes and shingles lesions. It does not kill the virus, but interrupts its replication by binding with the receptor sites needed by the virus to multiply. The essential oil is also included in perfume and massage oils.

Lemongrass (*Cymbopogon citratus*) is a member of the Poaceae (Grass) Family. The leaves are an important antioxidant, aromatic, antiseptic, and astringent. Lemongrass is used for oily and acne-prone skin and skin infections in the form of facial steams, cleansers, toners, lotions, soaps, and as a bath herb. Lemongrass is excellent for dandruff and oily hair and is used in shampoos, conditioners, and hair rinses. It also helps volumize the hair. The essential oil (also known as citronella) is used in deodorants and perfumery, and as a treatment for ringworm. The essential oil is also considered an antidepressant and helps promote mental alertness. Topically, lemongrass is used as a poultice for arthritis pain and a bath herb for sore muscles. It is added to massage oil to help backaches, sciatica, sprains, rheumatism, tendonitis, and varicose veins, and to improve circulation and muscle tone. It is used as a natural insect repellent against fleas, flies, and mosquitoes. The fresh herb can also be crushed and rubbed on the skin for the same effect.

Licorice root (*Glycyrrhiza glabra*, *G. uralensis*) is a member of the Fabaceae (Pea) Family. It is one of the most commonly used herbs in traditional Chinese medicine because it harmonizes the effects of other herbs and enters all twelve meridians, helping to prolong their effects. Licorice helps to induce feelings of calmness, peace, and harmony. Licorice is valued for its anti-inflammatory, antimutagenic, antioxidant, antiseptic, antispasmodic, demulcent, emollient, rejuvenative, and tonic properties. It can be used in washes, lotions, and salves for inflamed eyelids, dry eyes, eczema, herpes, itchy skin, psoriasis, rashes, shingles, and wounds. It is added to hair rinses to treat hair loss and dandruff. Licorice makes a soothing bath herb for eczema and psoriasis. It is included in mouthwashes for tooth decay prevention, gingivitis, and mouth sores. Licorice root has a soothing, detoxifying effect and helps prevent allergic reactions from other cosmetic ingredients. Licorice, the great harmonizer!

Linden (*Tilia species*) is a member of the Tiliaceae (Tilia) Family. The flowers are used cosmetically for their antiseptic, sedative, and vulnerary qualities. They are included in facial waters, facial steams, masks, lotions, moisturizers, and soaps. Linden helps leave the skin smooth and soft and minimizes wrinkles. It helps heal blood vessel walls and is used to clear acne, boils, burns, freckles, and rashes. Linden is included in shampoos, conditioners, and hair rinses. As a bath herb, it promotes relaxation. It can be used as a gargle for mouth sores. Take a walk in the springtime with a beloved one, underneath the linden flowers!

Loofah (*L. acutangula* and *L. aegyptiaca*) belongs to the Cucurbitaceae (Gourd) Family. A loofah is the dried skeleton of the gourd. Loofahs are exfoliating, and when used to scrub the skin, can help slough off dead skin cells. They are scratchy when dry and should be moistened before use. Be sure that the loofah dries out between uses to prevent bacterial proliferation. Loofahs are easy to grow and can be allowed to ripen on the vine until their skin turns dark yellow or brown. After collecting the gourds, soak them in a bucket of water to soften their skin. Peel off the skin, remove the seeds, and allow the loofahs to dry in the sun.

Lycii berries (*Lycium chinense*), also known as goji and wolfberry, help remove toxins from the blood by strengthening the kidneys and liver. They protect the liver against damage from toxin exposure. They have many other virtues, including being an aphrodisiac, a rejuvenative, and a tonic for the blood, energy, liver, and *yin* (fluids) of the body. They are a supreme eye food, helping to treat night blindness and blurred and poor vision. They are highly nutritive, containing beta-carotene, vitamins B_1, B_2, and C, and linoleic acid. Lycii are said to "brighten the spirit," and prolonged use promotes cheerfulness. Look for berries with a bright red color. Be sure that they have not been treated with sulfur. Eat them plain, like raisins, or add them to trail mix. They are also good mixed into a smoothie; soak them first to facilitate blending.

Macadamia nuts (*Macadamia tetraphylla*, *M. integrifolia*) are members of the Proteaceae (Protea) Family and also known as Queensland nuts. They are high in fat (70 percent) and low in protein (8 percent), but they also contain carbohydrates, calcium, iron, phosphorus, selenium, and zinc. The luxurious oil is easily absorbed into the skin and is useful in lotions and lip balms.

Mango (*Mangifera indica*) is a member of the Anacardiaceae (Cashew) Family. Mangoes are rich in amino acids, beta-carotene, niacin, vitamins C and E, flavonoids, calcium, iron, magnesium, and potassium. Some people are allergic to mangoes, especially the juice under the peel.

Mango butter is cold pressed from the seeds of mango fruits. It is solid at room temperature and makes products such as soaps and lotions very emollient.

Marshmallow root (*Althea officinalis*) is a member of the Malvaceae (Malva) Family. The root is used in beauty care for its anti-inflammatory and emollient properties. It is used in dry and sensitive skin treatments, as a bath herb, and in facial steams, cleansers, moisturizers, lotions, soaps, wrinkle creams, and salves. It is particularly helpful for eczema, psoriasis, sunburn, windburn, and wounds. Marshmallow root is high in mucilaginous compounds, which have a soothing, healing quality upon the skin. Its soothing properties make it nourishing for dry hair, and it is used in shampoos, conditioners, and hair rinses. Marshmallow is very drawing as well as soothing. The leaves and root are used as a poultice or compress to soothe burns, irritated eyes, mastitis, sunburn, varicose veins, and wounds. Eat freely of the wild garden herb *Malva neglecta*. It is fresh, free, and abundant, moistening your body with its essence and minerals.

Meadowsweet (*Filipendula ulmaria*) is a member of the Rosaceae (Rose) Family. The above-ground portions are used for their anti-inflammatory and aromatic properties. Meadowsweet is used as an eyewash for sore eyes and as a compress for rheumatism. The flowers are used to make facial steams and facial water to clear and brighten the complexion. The oil from the buds is used in perfumery.

Mullein (*Verbascum thapsus*) is a member of the Scrophulariaceae (Figwort) Family. The leaves are used for their astringent and emollient properties, and as a bath herb for sore muscles. The flowers are included in cosmetics such as facial creams for their softening properties, and as a hair rinse to highlight blonde hair. Mullein flower oil is used to treat bruises, sore muscles, hemorrhoids, and ringworm.

Myrrh resin (*Commiphora myrrha*) is a member of the Burseraceae (Frankincense) Family. Myrrh is valued for its analgesic, anti-inflammatory, antifungal, antiseptic, aromatic, rejuvenative, and vulnerary properties. Myrrh is an important infection-fighting agent and is included in salves to treat acne, boils, eczema, impetigo, ringworm, and varicose veins. It helps to promote tissue granulation and is therefore used in antiwrinkle creams. It is widely used in dental products, such as toothpastes and mouthwashes, to treat halitosis, mouth sores, thrush, gingivitis, pyorrhea, and cavities. Myrrh is used in soaps and as a fixative for perfumes to make them long-lasting; it is probably best known as incense. It is such a powerful preservative that it was used by the ancient Egyptians to make mummies. With so many uses, it's no wonder the wise men brought this gift from the East to the Christ child!

Neem (*Azadirachta indica*) is a member of the Meliaceae (Mahogany) Family. The bark, twigs, leaves, roots, seeds, and sap are valued for their antibacterial, antifungal, anti-inflammatory, antiseptic, antiviral, and pediculocide (lice-killing) properties. It is used in soaps, salves, and lotions to treat skin conditions such as acne, athlete's foot, eczema, rashes, ringworm, scabies, wounds, and even leprosy. As a bath herb, neem helps chicken pox and rashes. Juice from the leaves is applied to boils and eczema. Twigs of neem are used as toothbrushes to prevent gum disease, treat gingivitis, and prevent plaque buildup. The oil is used to condition hair, treat dandruff, and deter head lice. When added to nail care products, it helps prevent splitting and breakage. Neem is added to cosmetics as a natural preservative as well as to benefit many skin conditions. Neem is an important plant globally, and could replace many harmful chemicals.

Neroli (*Citrus bigaradia*, *C. aurantium*) is a member of the Rutaceae (Citrus) Family. Neroli oil, from orange blossoms, is sweet and cooling; it relieves anxiety, stress, and grief. Neroli oil is used to rejuvenate and moisturize the skin. Neroli is considered antidepressant, aphrodisiac, sedative, and uplifting. Take a walk in a flowering orange grove and breathe deeply.

Nettle (*Urtica dioica*) is a member of the Urticaceae (Nettle) Family. The aboveground portions are used for their antifungal, astringent, nutritive, and stimulating properties. Nettle tea is an internal beauty herb and is excellent to strengthen hair, skin, and nails due to its high concentration of nutrients including calcium, iron, silica, sulfur, and beta-carotene. It is also used internally for the treatment of acne, boils, and eczema and to help improve circulation. Nettle's astringent and mineral-rich properties make it a tonic for the face, body, scalp, and hair. It helps to balance over-oily conditions and deters fungal and bacterial growth. Consumed regularly, it helps clear up dark circles under the eyes. Nettle is included in facial steams and cleansers, especially for oily skin. Nettle helps curb the appetite and cleanses toxins from the body. Since nettle is energizing, it helps in the motivation to stay on a healthful diet. My favorite health tonic is fresh nettle juice. It literally makes you feel high. My husband and I dig a daily dose. The rest of the year, we enjoy it as a regular infusion. Nettle is used in shampoos and conditioners to treat dandruff and hair loss, add shine, and naturally darken color. As nettle is acidic, it promotes shiny hair and helps prevent graying; it is an old Gypsy secret for luxurious and shiny locks. Nettle in a final hair rinse makes an excellent conditioner and helps normalize the sebaceous glands. Nettle helps control dandruff, even stubborn cases, when used internally and topically. Roots, leaves, and seeds are all used in hair preparations, including antidandruff shampoo. To treat hair loss, a tea, a tincture, or the juice of the leaves and roots of nettle can be rubbed daily into the scalp. This sounds wild, but throughout history, those with hair loss have stung their scalps with fresh nettle to increase circulation and promote hair growth. Nettle's high chlorophyll content makes the juice effective as a natural breath freshener. Nettle used in mouthwashes and toothpastes helps reduce plaque and gingivitis. Fresh nettle can cause a stinging rash reaction due to the presence of formic acid and histamine; however, the dried, puréed, or heated plant has no such effect. Even my kids, friends, and students know that getting stung with nettle is one of the most effective anti-cellulite treatments. Rudolph Steiner called nettle "the heart of the world."

Nutmeg (*Myristica fragrans*) is a member of the Myristicaceae (Nutmeg) Family. The kernels are used for their anti-inflammatory, aphrodisiac, astringent, and circulatory-stimulating properties. Nutmeg is incorporated into salves to treat eczema, ringworm, and scars. Nutmeg is added to hair rinses to stimulate hair growth. The essential oil of nutmeg is used in massage oils for muscular pain and in perfumes and soaps. It is said to help prevent scar formation. It can be applied to a toothache until dental assistance is available. It is also a popular ingredient in aftershaves. Nutmeg essential oil invigorates the brain, calms and strengthens the nerves, and has long been considered an aphrodisiac. Inhale some deeply as aromatherapy. (Ecstasy, "the love drug," was originally derived from sassafras and nutmeg.)

Oats (*Avena fatua*, *A. sativa*) belong to the Poaceae (Grass) Family. Use leftover oatmeal from breakfast as a mask or scrub for blackheads and/or dry, oily, or wrinkled skin. It helps soften the skin and can be used instead of soap as a cleansing agent for very sensitive skin. Oats are used in soaps, lotions, and sunscreens for their soothing and anti-inflammatory properties. Oat flakes are used topically as a bath herb to soften skin and to help itchy skin, eczema, hives, rheumatism, and neuralgia. Whole oats (oat groats) that have not been heated can be soaked and sprouted.

Olive oil (*Olea europaea*) is a member of the Oleaceae (Olive) Family. Made from pressing ripe olives, this rich oil is excellent for very dry, normal, sensitive, and sun-damaged skin. It is deeply penetrating and rich in vitamins and minerals. It is a good antioxidant due to its high vitamin E content. It is warming and excellent in cold weather and to improve muscular pain. It is also beneficial for abrasions, bruises, and burns. It blocks about 20 percent of UV rays. Olive oil is included in creams, lotions, conditioners, and soaps. Soaps with a large percentage of olive oil are often labeled as "castile" soap. Be sure to use extra-virgin olive oil, which is from the first pressing and the most nutritious.

After the first pressing, chemical solvents may be used to extract the oil. It is shelf stable, does not easily turn rancid, and is effective and inexpensive.

Orange flower water (*Citrus species*) is derived from a member of the Rutaceae (Citrus) Family. Spritz it on dry skin and broken capillaries to stimulate new cell growth. It is also incorporated into perfumes. Orange oil is anti-inflammatory and sedative. Share oranges with your comrades. Be one with the fruits.

Oregon grape (*Mahonia repens*) is a member of the Berberidaceae (Barberry) Family. The root and root bark are primarily used internally for their antiseptic properties to treat conditions such as acne, boils, eczema, herpes, and impetigo. It is made into a salve for itchy skin, boils, wounds, and various skin infections.

Orrisroot (*Iris florentina*) is a member of the Iridaceae (Iris) Family. Orrisroot is considered a fixative and helps other herbs retain their scent when mixed together. For this reason, it is an important ingredient in sachets and potpourris. The juice of the plant is applied to the skin to lighten freckles. The powdered root is used to make dry shampoos. The roots are also chewed as a breath freshener. The essential oil has a fragrance reminiscent of violets, due to the presence of the ketone irone and is used to scent toothpastes, soaps, and powders. My husband, bless his heart, naturally smells like orrisroot.

Palmarosa (*Cymbopogon martini*) is a member of the Poaceae (Grass) Family. Its essential oil is used topically in lotions to treat acne and psoriasis. It is considered antibacterial. In aromatherapy, it is used to comfort grief, and relieve possessiveness.

Panthenol is also known as vitamin B_5 or pantothenic acid. It is one of the B vitamins that is used to prevent graying of the hair. It is added to hair sprays, styling gels, and shampoos to add body to the hair.

Papaya (*Carica papaya*) is rich in antioxidants, especially vitamin C and beta-carotene. When consumed regularly, papaya improves the health of the skin, hair, nails, and eyes. Papain powder (made from dried juice of the green fruit) is applied to bee stings to reduce pain and inflammation; it is also used as a tooth and gum cleanser. Papaya leaves are used as a poultice for wounds. The unripe fruit is used in exfoliating facial masks to nourish the skin, improve oily skin, lighten freckles, and heal scars. Green papaya is even more effective, as there are more enzymes present in the unripe fruit.

Parsley (*Petroselinum crispum*) is a member of the Apiaceae (Parsley) Family. The leaves are valued for their antioxidant, antiseptic, and nutritive qualities. Eating parsley on a regular basis helps to promote clear skin and is a Gypsy favorite food for the eyes. In the Jewish tradition, parsley symbolizes new beginnings. Munching parsley at the end of a meal is an instant sugar-free breath freshener. A parsley mask can help blackheads, blotchy skin, and troubled complexions. Parsley is a welcome addition to facial steams for dry and oily skin. It is used in lotions for its soothing properties and can help eczema and psoriasis. It can be used in compresses to soothe tired eyes. It is included in hair rinses for dark hair and to treat dandruff. As a mouthwash, it helps to freshen the breath. The essential oil from the seed is used in perfumery.

Patchouli leaves (*Pogostemon patchouli*, *P. cablin*) are members of the Lamiaceae (Mint) Family. Well known for its scent, the leaves are aged for at least twenty-four hours before being distilled. The essential oil is considered antifungal, aphrodisiac, antiseptic, deodorant, and rejuvenative. It is used in cleansers, moisturizers, soaps, and salves to treat acne, athlete's foot, eczema, and dry, mature skin. It is used in shampoos, conditioners, and hair rinses for the treatment of dandruff. Patchouli calms anxiety, lifts the spirits, stimulates the nervous system, improves clarity, and attracts sexual love. Fabrics, including rugs and shawls, imported from India are impregnated with the smell of patchouli as a moth deterrent.

Peach (*Prunus persica*, *P. vulgaris*) belongs to the Rosaceae (Rose) Family. In the Taoist tradition, peaches are considered a fruit of immortality and to this day are consumed for longevity. Eat peaches to improve skin tone, promote circulation, and reduce excess perspiration. Peaches are cool, sweet and sour, and antioxidant. They are high in beta-carotene, vitamin C, calcium, boron, magnesium, phosphorus, potassium, and flavonoids. Used as a facial mask, peaches enliven tired skin and deter wrinkles. The pulverized seeds are used as an exfoliant.

Peanut (*Arachis hypogaea*) is not a nut at all but a member of the Fabaceae (Pea) Family. Peanuts slow metabolism, can inhibit thyroid function, and are a common allergen. They are often contaminated with a mold called aflatoxin that is produced by a fungus (*Aspergillus flavus*), which is considered a carcinogen. Peanuts are hard to digest and are especially difficult on the liver. Peanuts can aggravate skin breakouts like acne and eczema, and excess consumption can promote lethargy and obesity. Peanut fields are often rotated with cotton, which is a heavily sprayed crop. Peanut oil is used topically for dry skin; it is deeply penetrating and has a fairly stable shelf life. Use it with caution, as it can be a severe allergen for some people.

Pear (*Pyrus communis*) is a member of the Rosaceae (Rose) Family. Pears are cool, sweet, and mildly sour. Pears are a good source of beta-carotene, folic acid, and vitamin C. As a facial, pears benefit dry, normal, and oily skin. They calm inflamed, blotchy skin and sunburn. Pears, roses, and apples are all governed by Venus, goddess of love and beauty.

Peppermint (*Mentha piperita*) is a very aromatic member of the Lamiaceae (Mint) Family. It is a cooling and stimulating antiseptic and antiviral. It is a refreshing and stimulating ingredient in baths, soaps, facial steams, masks, toners, aftershaves, shampoos, conditioners, and hair rinses. Peppermint is also used for its breath-freshening properties in toothpastes and mouthwashes. It makes an invigorating and deodorizing footbath. **Spearmint** (*Mentha spicata*) can be used as a scrub for dry, tight skin. It dissolves as you scrub, protecting the skin from being abraded. Spearmint is similar to peppermint but with a lower menthol content; thus it is less medicinal smelling and somewhat sweeter and lighter.

Persimmon (*Diospyros virginiana*, *D. kaki*) is a member of the Ebenaceae (Ebony) Family. They are high in beta-carotene and used as a facial mask for all skin types. They lubricate the lungs, strengthen the spleen and pancreas, improve energy, and contain enzymes that help break down damaged cells and foreign microbes.

Petitgrain (*Citrus aurantium*), a member of the Rutaceae (Citrus) Family, is derived from orange leaves. It is antibacterial, anti-inflammatory, and calming. It is sometimes referred to as "poor man's neroli." On an emotional level, it is used to calm panic and anxiety.

Pine (*Pinus species*) is a member of the Pinaceae (Pine) Family. Aromatic and antiseptic, pine is cooling, astringent, anti-inflammatory, and stimulating. Pine is valued as a bath herb for sore muscles and is used in soaps, lotions, perfumes, and aftershaves. Pine helps remedy acne, eczema, and psoriasis when used in soaps and lotions. Pine is used in salves to treat eczema and psoriasis and to bring boils to a head. Pine is also incorporated into antidandruff shampoos, conditioners, and hair rinses. Take a walk in a pine forest and take in the sweet and pungent green energy.

Pineapple (*Anana comosus*) is a member of the Bromeliaceae (Pineapple) Family. Pineapple is cooling and moist and helps the skin retain youthfulness. Pineapple is antibacterial, antiviral, and demulcent. The fresh fruit contains the enzyme bromelain, which helps digest protein and reduce inflammation. The alpha hydroxy acids dissolve the bond that holds dead skin cells together; thus it is exfoliating and helps diminish wrinkles, scars, and warts when applied topically. A small amount can be used to wash your face instead of soap.

Plantain (*Plantago major*) is a member of the Plantaginaceae (Plantain) Family. The leaves are valued for their antiseptic, anti-inflammatory, astringent, demulcent, mucilaginous, and refrigerant properties. It is a superb herb containing allantoin, which is used in salves to promote tissue repair, draw out toxins, soothe wounds, and repair damaged, wrinkled skin. It can be used as a hair rinse for dandruff and a douche for vaginitis. It is used as a bath herb for dry skin. Plantain promotes tissue repair and soothes irritated mucous membranes. It is employed as a poultice for toothaches and as a salve for bleeding, bee stings, boils, bruises, burns, eczema, hemorrhoids, insect bites, mastitis, poison ivy/oak, ringworm, snakebites, splinters, sunburn, ulcers, and wounds. It is such a hardy plant it grows through the cracks in sidewalks.

Psyllium (*Plantago psyllium*, *P. ovata*) is a member of the Plantaginaceae (Plantain) Family. The seeds and outer husk of seeds are employed as a laxative and stool softener. They are traditionally used to treat constipation and obesity. One teaspoon is taken in a bit of water or juice to curb hunger by causing a feeling of fullness in the stomach and to promote normal elimination. Drink the mixture quickly before it gels. It can also be taken in capsules. Psyllium is high in mucilage and essential fatty acids. The seeds absorb about eight to fourteen times their weight in water. Their fibrous quality makes them laxative, yet they also provide intestinal bulk, which can stop diarrhea. Because they tend to swell and create a feeling of fullness, they can help curb appetite. Always use psyllium with plenty of liquids; otherwise, it can *cause* constipation. Psyllium can dilute digestive enzymes and is best taken between meals—especially before bed or first thing upon rising—rather than with food.

Pumice stone is cooled lava rock containing mostly silicates. It is very porous and rough to the touch. It is most often used on the feet but can also be rubbed on the knees, elbows, and hands. Pumice stones work best when wet; soak your stone for three to five minutes, and soak your feet in warm water for about fifteen minutes before using a pumice stone on them. Avoid sharing your stone with others. Allow your pumice stone to dry fully between uses to deter bacterial growth.

Pumpkin (*Cucurbita pepo*) is a member of the Cucurbitaceae (Gourd) Family. Being rich in beta-carotene, they improve skin health. Pumpkins are antioxidant and benefit conditions such as acne and eczema. Raw pumpkin contains enzymes that exfoliate the skin and have anti-inflammatory properties. Native Americans have long used mashed pumpkin as a soothing topical application for abscesses, boils, bruises, burns, and sprains.

Red clover flowers and leaves (*Trifolium pratense*) belong to the Fabaceae (Pea) Family. They are valued for their alterative, antibacterial, anti-inflammatory, emollient, and vulnerary properties. Red clover is used internally to help clear skin conditions such as acne, eczema, and psoriasis. It is included in facial steams, cleansers, lotions, and moisturizers. It is also used as a bath herb for many skin conditions including acne, eczema, psoriasis, and sun and wind damage. It is included in lip balms for its soothing properties. Red clover is included in shampoos, conditioners, and hair rinses for dry or damaged hair. Red clover cleanses and clears toxins, nourishes and moves the blood, and stimulates lymphatic movement. It reduces swelling and inflammation, reduces respiratory irritation, and promotes tissue repair. Red clover is used as a poultice, compress, salve, or wash for athlete's foot, arthritic pain, burns, skin cancer, eczema, gout, insect bites, lymphatic swelling, psoriasis, tumors, and wounds.

Red palm oil (*Elaesis guineensis*) is a member of the Palmaceae (Palm) Family. It is used in Africa the same way that people in Mediterranean countries use olive oil. The oil is red or orange in color and is high in beta-carotene and vitamin E. It is shelf stable.

Rose (*Rosa species*) is a member of the Rosaceae (Rose) Family. The flowers are used in body care for their antiseptic, aromatic, astringent, hydrating, rejuvenative, and soothing properties. Rose is beloved for its beautiful scent and as an ingredient for dry and mature skin in facial steams, cleansers, lotions, toners, moisturizers, and bath products. Rose is considered a cell rejuvenator. For dry hair, roses are included in shampoos, conditioners, and hair rinses. Rose flowers are used in cosmetics to smooth and soften dry, wrinkled skin. Roses make a delightfully fragrant bath addition and a good poultice for swellings. Rose hip seed oil is high in essential fatty acids and is excellent for skin regeneration and scar prevention and helps reduce the appearance of wrinkles. Rose water, made by distillation, soothes and opens the heart chakra; it is wonderful for dry skin, bruises, sprains, and pulled muscles, and is used as a compress for sore eyes and conjunctivitis. Rose water can be sprinkled on the forehead to cool a fever; during medieval times, it was used to treat insanity. Diluted, it is applied to cotton balls and placed on closed eyes to reduce puffiness. Rose water makes a lovely, cool, refreshing facial spray and mouthwash. Pure rose essential oil is one of the most wonderful and expensive scents and is commonly included in perfumery. Before you balk at the price of pure rose oil, be aware that it takes 180 pounds of rose blossoms to make just one ounce of the essential oil, about 10,000 pounds of roses to make 1 pound of the essential oil, and 30 roses to make 1 drop of oil. Rose essential oil is used in skin care products for acne, dryness, and wrinkles. Rose is considered sacred to Aphrodite (Venus) and is the queen of all flowers. Rose is associated with physical and spiritual love and is a supreme heart opener. Rose is both sensual and romantic and helps heal grief from emotional trauma. Rose flowers are used medicinally to treat anger, anxiety, depression, and grief. Roses are good for anyone who feels distanced from his or her emotional center. When you want to rekindle the spark of love, use rose oil while making love. Place one diluted drop on your forehead before sleep to have dreams of love. Place a drop of rose oil on your and your lover's heart chakras after first smelling it.

Rosemary (*Rosmarinus officinalis*) is a member of the Lamiaceae (Mint) Family. Frequent smelling of rosemary is beautifying. *Banck's Herbal* (1525) advises, "Smell it oft and it shall keep you youngly." The leaves are antioxidant, antiseptic, astringent, rejuvenative, and stimulating. When used on the skin, it helps to strengthen the capillaries and improve sluggish and mature wrinkled skin. It is widely used in facial steams, cleansers, masks, toners, lotions, moisturizers, and soaps. It is an ingredient in Queen of Hungary Water (see page 48), a popular beauty tonic. As a bath herb, rosemary relaxes sore muscles while keeping the mind alert. Rosemary is included in salves for bruises, eczema, sprains, and rheumatism. It is made into a gargle for sore throat, gum ailments, and canker sores, and is used to freshen the breath. It makes a stimulating eyewash. Sachets of dried rosemary are placed in one's pillowcase to stimulate dreams and prevent nightmares. Rosemary is popular in hair products, such as shampoos, conditioners, and rinses, to help darken gray hair, remove excess oils, treat dandruff, and deter hair loss. Add a few drops of rosemary essential oil after washing your hairbrush to impart a beautiful shine and fragrance to your hair and stimulate growth. It is included in toothpastes and mouthwashes and is used as an insect repellent. Rosemary essential oil is a rubefacient and is used as a liniment for neuralgia, sciatica, cellulite, and sore muscles. Inhalation of rosemary essential oil is used to improve memory and Alzheimer's disease, calm anxiety, and prevent fainting. Almost every holiday season, my family and friends make rosemary dream pillows to give away and use ourselves.

Rosewood (*Aniba rosaeodora*) is a member of the Lauraceae (Laurel) Family. It is a valuable rain-forest resource. It can be an important cell rejuvenative agent, beneficial for all skin types. It is also used in aromatherapy as an antidepressant and to encourage tranquility. Too many rosewood trees have been cut, and thus they need to be protected. Coriander essential oil can be used as a substitute.

Safflower (*Carthamus tinctorius*) is a member of the Asteraceae (Daisy) Family. The flowers are used as an analgesic, antibacterial, anticoagulant, anti-inflammatory, vasodilator, and vulnerary. Topically, safflowers are used as a liniment for bruises, sprains, and inflammations, as they stimulate tissue regeneration. They are used to color cosmetics red, such as rouge, and to make yellow and red dye for fabric. The oil, made from the seeds, is high in linoleic acid and is used for massage and in body care products such as lotions for normal to oily skin. It is also used in hair-growth preparations in Asia. It is widely used, as it is inexpensive.

Sage (*Salvia officinalis*) is a member of the Lamiaceae (Mint) Family. The leaves and flowers are antibacterial, astringent, and antiseptic, and are included in skin care products such as facial steams, cleansers, toners, and soaps. It is also used as a bath herb. Sage is especially beneficial for acne and oily skin. It has been used as a wash and salve to treat eczema, psoriasis, and poison oak and ivy. A poultice of fresh sage leaves is used for insect bites and wounds. Sage is very effective as an antiperspirant when included in deodorants. It is a common ingredient in shampoos, conditioners, and rinses for oily hair, hair loss, brunette hair, and to darken gray hair. It helps to stimulate the scalp. Sage is breath freshening when added to toothpastes and mouthwashes, and helps treat gingivitis. The fresh leaves are rubbed on teeth as a whitening agent. Sage makes an excellent gargle for mouth sores, laryngitis, sore throat, sore gums, and tonsillitis. The dried herb is burned as incense for purification of negative energy. Here is an ancient saying about sage (which I've also heard said about gotu kola): "Eating a few sage leaves a day will keep old age away."

Salt (sodium chloride) is best when it is unrefined and not bleached white. The wetter, grayer types of salt, such as Celtic sea salt, contain trace minerals. Salt is antiseptic and astringent. Salt is drying, drawing, cleansing, and abrasive. It is used in body scrubs, tooth powders, and in baths. It helps relieve itching and improves poison ivy and athlete's foot.

Sandalwood (*Santalum album*) is a member of the Santalaceae (Sandalwood) Family. Sandalwood is antiseptic, aphrodisiac, astringent, and rejuvenative. It calms skin irritations in conditions such as chapped dry skin and eczema and is used as a bath herb. It is added to shampoos, conditioners, and hair rinses. The essential oil is a common ingredient in exotic perfumes and colognes, with a history of 4,000 years of use. In many tropical places, women mix sandalwood essential oil with coconut oil and rub it into their hair for a beautiful shine and fragrance. Sandalwood is used as a base for most woodsy perfumes. Its chemistry is similar to androsterone, one of the male hormones. Sandalwood essential oil is massaged into the forehead for its calming effects and to enhance meditation. When inhaled, it can uplift depression and improve fatigue and coughs. Sandalwood is used to scent soaps, lotions, and aftershaves. Sandalwood trees take at least twenty-five years to grow. In order for the essential oil to be made, the tree needs to be cut down, which is contributing to the decimation of sandalwood trees and the high cost. Either leave this herb alone or only use sustainably harvested products.

Sangre del Grado (*Croton lechleri*) is a resin from a plant in the Euphorbiaceae (Spurge) Family. It is also known as "dragon's blood." It is taken internally and used topically to stop bleeding, seal and heal wounds, and treat insect bites and viral infections, such as herpes, as well as fungal overgrowth, such as athlete's foot. It is antiseptic and a vulnerary.

Sarsaparilla (*Smilax officinalis*) is a member of the Smilaceae (Smilax) Family. It is used internally for its alterative, diaphoretic, and rejuvenative properties to remedy skin concerns such as acne, age spots, eczema, and psoriasis. It helps reduce inflammation by binding with bacteria and carrying it out of the body.

Sea buckthorn (*Hippophaë rhamnoides*) is a member of the Elaeagnaceae (Oleaster) Family. The genus name *Hippophaë* means "shiny horse" in Greek and refers to the shiny coat that horses develop after feeding on this herb. Sea buckthorn has been fed to racehorses and in mythology was said to have been the preferred food of flying horses, such as Pegasus. The ripe berries are used as an analgesic, antibiotic, anti-inflammatory, antioxidant, and tonic. The berries are seven times higher in vitamin C than lemons. They are also rich in beta-carotene, lycopene, and essential fatty acids. Sea buckthorn is used topically on the skin in the form of oils, salves, balms, and lotions to treat acne, burns, dermatitis, eczema, infections, and wrinkles, and to prevent sunburn. Russian cosmonauts have used this herb for radiation burns when in outer space. After the disaster at the nuclear power plant in Chernobyl, sea buckthorn oil was used to treat the radiation burns of people exposed. Sea buckthorn is used in hair products to prevent baldness and stimulate hair growth. It is often planted to help prevent soil erosion and can be replanted in areas that have been damaged by mining. It also provides food and shelter for many animals.

Sesame oil is good for dry, normal, and oily skin. It is used in sunscreen preparations, as it blocks about 30 percent of the sun's rays. It has a long shelf life, and it washes out of fabrics more easily than other oils.

Sesame seeds (*Sesamum indicum*) belong to the Pedaliaceae (Sesame) Family. The seeds are about 50 percent oil and 25–35 percent protein. They also contain vitamin E, calcium, iron, and sesamin, a lignin that is a powerful antioxidant. The seeds are considered demulcent, emollient, laxative, and a general tonic. They strengthen bones, hair, nails, and teeth. Black sesame seeds are used in Asian medicine to prevent hair from graying and to tonify the kidneys.

Shea butter comes from the shea tree (*Vitellaria paradoxa, Butyrospermum parkii*), which is native to Africa. It is also known as karite butter or African butter. It is rich in beta-carotene and vitamin E. It increases local capillary circulation, helps heal bruising, and acts as a deeply penetrating and rich moisturizer for dry skin. It is included in soaps, lotions, and sunscreens and is beneficial for eczema, psoriasis, stretch marks, and wounds. It contains a plant sterol known as stigmasterol that helps reduce stiffness and is included in creams and massage oils for stiff arthritic joints. It does offer some sun protection factor—about SPF 6, blocking about 30 percent of ultraviolet radiation. Its high linoleic acid content makes it excellent for soothing chapped, burned, or irritated skin. Shea butter solidifies at around 70 degrees F and liquefies when warmer. When applied daily, it helps to soften and lighten age spots.

Soapwort root (*Saponaria officinalis*) is a member of the Caryophyllaceae (Pink) Family. When mixed with water, it produces a foamy lather, due to its saponin content. Soapwort can be used as a wash to clean the body. When used as a shampoo, it imparts softness and shininess and brings out highlights. It helps to effectively remove grease and has long been used to wash clothes.

Southernwood leaves (*Artemisia abrotanum*) belongs to the Asteraceae (Daisy) Family. It is used as a remedy against hair loss. It is sometimes mixed with olive oil and used as a hot oil treatment for dry hair. When used as a hair rinse, it brings out highlights.

Soybean (*Glycine max*) from the Fabaceae (Pea) Family is high in linoleic acid, lecithin, and vitamin E. As a food plant, though high in protein, it is a common allergen and can be difficult for many to digest unless in a fermented form, such as unpasteurized tempeh, miso or tamari. When used as an oil and applied topically, it can clog pores.

Star anise (*Illicium verum*) is a member of the Magnoliaceae (Magnolia) Family. The fruits are valued for their analgesic, aromatic, and circulatory-stimulating properties. The essential oil is used to scent hair products, soaps, and perfume. Chew a small piece after a meal to freshen your breath.

Strawberry fruit (*Fragaria virginiana*) is a member of the Rosaceae (Rose) Family. Crushed berries are exfoliating and are applied on the skin as a mask to relieve sunburn, lighten freckles, tighten pores, and improve oily and blemished skin. Strawberries are rubbed over the teeth to whiten them and remove plaque, without damaging dental enamel.

Sugar comes from either sugarcane (*Saccharum officinarum*) or beets (*Beta vulgaris*). It takes one yard of sugarcane to make one teaspoon of sugar. Sugar can be used as an exfoliating scrub. It is gentle because it dissolves before causing abrasion. Eliminating sugar as a food is essential for ultimate beauty. Get your sweet treats from fresh fruits and vegetables.

Sunflower (*Helianthus annuus*) is a member of the Asteraceae (Daisy) Family. As a medicinal food, sunflower seeds are considered antioxidant, diuretic, expectorant, nutritive, and warming. They decrease light sensitivity and prevent eye degeneration. They strengthen the fingernails due to their high nutrient content. Rich in polyunsaturated fatty acids, vitamin E, lecithin, and linoleic acid, sunflower oil can be used as massage oil for normal and dry skin and rheumatic limbs.

Talc, made from powdered soapstone, has been linked to ovarian and lung cancers and should not be inhaled. It is still used on babies, added to makeup, and included as filler in cosmetic creams, though it is not recommended. If you want to use a powder, look for one that is based on arrowroot, rice powder, or cornstarch.

Tea (*Camellia sinensis*) is a member of the Theaceae (Tea) Family. It helps prevent dental decay by inhibiting the enzyme *Streptococcus mutans*, which is responsible for plaque formation. Tea contains carotenoids, chlorophyll, caffeine, theophylline, theobromine, gamma-aminobutyric acid, polysaccharides, fats, vitamins C and E, manganese, potassium, zinc, and fluoride. A cup of green tea a day has been found to decrease cavities by half in children. It can also help inhibit the bacteria that causes halitosis. Green tea is traditionally consumed after a meal to leave the mouth feeling fresh and clean. Lukewarm green tea has even been used topically on open wounds, acne, athlete's foot, and sunburn. Green tea, when used topically, appears to protect the skin from damage from ultraviolet radiation exposure and may reduce the incidence of skin cancer due to its antioxidant activity. Green tea is diuretic and thermogenic. It prevents the blood from "clumping together" and forming clots that can lead to stroke. The catechin content of green tea helps to break down cholesterol and increase its elimination through the bowels. Green tea also helps to keep blood sugar levels moderate and promotes clarity and energy. Even though caffeine gets a bad rap, the caffeine in green tea increases the syntheses of catecholamines, which are stimulant chemicals that relay nerve impulses in the brain. Green tea has about 25 mg of caffeine per cup (black tea has 35–40). The caffeine content of green tea is about as much as a soda and one-third to half as much as a cup of coffee. The tannins also help to preserve the body's own storehouse of vitamin C. Excessive use of green tea can cause nervous irritability and aggravate ulcers. Avoid it in cases of hypertension and insomnia.

Tea tree (*Melaleuca alternifolia*) is a member of the Myrtaceae (Eucalyptus) Family. The essential oil is distilled from the leaves and is an excellent antifungal and antiseptic agent. The oil is added to facial steams, cleansers, soaps, toners, lotions, moisturizers, and salves, and is added to the bath. It helps skin conditions such as acne, eczema, and psoriasis, and also fights fungal infections such as diaper rash, jock itch, ringworm, and athlete's foot. It is an excellent insect repellent and can deter mosquitoes, fleas, ticks, and even scabies. Tea tree oil is also used in shampoos, conditioners, and hair rinses, and can help dandruff and even prevent head lice. Combs and brushes can be soaked in a solution of one pint alcohol with three drops of tea tree oil to help delouse hair care tools. The oil is effective when applied directly to pimples, cuts, bites, and warts. It has been used to protect the skin from radiation burns during cancer therapy. It is nonirritating and is one of the few essential oils, besides lavender, that can be applied directly to the skin without being diluted. For nail fungus, the affected area is soaked in undiluted tea tree oil twice daily.

Thyme (*Thymus vulgaris*) is a member of the Lamiaceae (Mint) Family. The leaves and flowers are antiseptic, aromatic, astringent, and stimulating. It is so powerful that during World War I thyme was used to disinfect soldiers' wounds. Thyme is included in facial steams, masks, cleansers, toners, soaps, deodorants, and aftershave products, and it is used as a bath herb. It helps treat acne, eczema, and psoriasis, and it is especially beneficial for oily skin conditions. In shampoos, conditioners, and hair rinses, thyme helps darken the hair, keeping it dandruff free and silky. The essential oil is added to massage oils for sore muscles and has been applied topically for warts. It is used in antifungal preparations, such as salves and washes, to deter athlete's foot, ringworm, scabies, crabs, and lice. It is used in mouthwashes for its antiseptic properties and to prevent plaque formation. The essential oil can be irritating to some skin types.

Tomato (*Lycopersicon esculentum*) is a member of the Solanaceae (Nightshade) Family. When used as a facial, tomato refines pores, decreases blackheads, and works as an exfoliant. Tomato is good for dry, blemished, and oily skin, and helps to restore the natural acid balance of the skin.

Tragacanth gum (*Astragalus gummifer*) is a member of the Fabaceae (Pea) Family. This gumlike resin, obtained from the root and stem of a spiny shrub, is used as a thickening agent for lotions, moisturizers, hairstyling gels, mascaras, eye shadows, foundations, and toothpastes. It is rich in mucilage and very demulcent. It was once burned as an incense to fumigate clothing and homes.

Tuberose (*Polianthes tuberosa*) is a member of the Amaryllidaceae (Amaryllis) Family. Available as an absolute, it is used in floral and Asian perfumes for its sweet, cooling, and floral scent. Considered an antidepressant and aphrodisiac, tuberose strengthens and evokes the emotions.

Turmeric root (*Curcuma longa*) is a member of the Zingiberaceae (Ginger) Family. In Asian medicine, turmeric is consumed to promote a softer and healthier complexion. It is an excellent anti-inflammatory agent and antioxidant. Turmeric can be sprinkled on a bleeding wound to stop the flow. It makes an excellent poultice for sunburned skin. In a salve, it helps relieve eczema and psoriasis. It is used in facial masks to beautify the skin. Add one teaspoon of turmeric to one cup of hot water to highlight blonde and light brown hair. It can stain clothing, so be careful!

Vanilla (*Vanilla planifolia*) is a member of the Orchidaceae (Orchid) Family. The cured seedpods are valued in cosmetics for their aphrodisiac and aromatic

Cosmetics and Chemistry

All cosmetic ingredients, whether natural or synthetic, are indeed made from chemicals. And some products, though originally from nature, have been synthesized. However, some come from nature and some come from polluting factories. The most damaging ingredients in skin and hair care products may cause skin sensitivity or eye irritation:

- Artificial colors are usually derived from coal tar or petroleum by-products.
- Collagen and elastin are proclaimed as "wonder drugs" by the cosmetic industry. However, they are made of animal bones and hooves or derived through the extraction of slaughtered animal wastes, tendons, cartilage, and skin. Think about it.
- Foaming agents that create lots of lather, including those in toothpastes, shampoos, and bath additives, can attack natural skin flora, causing it to become more brittle and dry and leading to a need for even more moisturizers.
- Synthetic sunscreens, including benzophenone-3 and octyl methoxycinnamate (OMC), can accumulate in breast milk and exhibit estrogenic effects.
- "Coc," "laur," and "myr" usually indicate emulsifiers. They may be derived from coconut or possibly from tallow (beef fat).
- Nitrosamines, also listed as DEA, TEA, and MEA, are suspected carcinogens. DEA is readily absorbed through the skin, accumulates in the organs, and is considered a cancer risk. It is commonly included in

qualities. Vanilla bean is often included in lotions, moisturizers, soaps, and perfumes. Because the plant must now be hand pollinated, due to the extinction of a particular bee caused by pesticide use, vanilla is the second most-expensive herb in the world. Available as an absolute or oleoresin, vanilla calms the emotions and appeases anger and irritability. Vanilla is considered the most sensual fragrance by older men; it is also enjoyed by babies who perhaps find it a close scent to mother's milk. It is believed that the smell of vanilla may stimulate the release of the neurotransmitter serotonin, triggering feelings of arousal and satisfaction.

Vervain herb (*Verbena officinalis*) is a member of the Verbenaceae (Verbena) Family. It is used in body care for its anti-inflammatory, astringent, vasoconstrictor, and vulnerary properties. Salves and poultices of the herb are used to remedy bruises, burns, eczema, hemorrhoids, and wounds. It is used in tonic hair rinses as a restorative for hair loss. The powdered herb is used as a tooth cleanser and is added to mouthwashes to treat gum disease and prevent cavities.

Vetivert (*Vetiveria zizanoides*) is a member of the Poaceae (Grass) Family. Its roots are distilled into an essential oil that is used is skin creams to treat acne, dryness, and wounds. It improves circulation, and when used topically, eases muscular pain. Its scent is uplifting yet calming. It is used in modern perfumery as a fixative.

Vinegar, especially apple cider vinegar, is included as a cosmetic ingredient because it is astringent, deodorizing, and antifungal. It can be used in place of alcohol in making tinctures. Vinegar is also made from grapes and rice. All vinegars contain between 4 and 6 percent acetic acid. Vinegar improves circulation and is inexpensive. It helps rinse calcium residue and soap out of hair, fights dandruff and oily hair, cleanses blemishes, cools sunburn, and exfoliates dead and oily skin. Excellent in aftershaves, vinegar helps restore an acidic pH after shampooing. I prefer raw apple cider vinegar. Vinegar can irritate open sores and sensitive skin.

Violet (*Viola odorata*) is a member of the Violaceae (Violet) Family. The leaves and flowers are antiseptic, astringent, demulcent, and nutritive. Used internally, they help to clear the skin of acne, boils, eczema, and psoriasis. Topically, they are excellent for dry, normal, and oily skin, and are included in facial steams, cleansers, toners, lotions, moisturizers, and as a bath herb. The leaves can be used as a compress or eyewash for sore eyes. Eat fresh leaves to improve visual and audial acuity and to prevent cancer.

Vitamin C (ascorbic acid) is added to skin creams as an antioxidant, antiaging nutrient, and preservative. In the body, vitamin C is necessary for collagen production and to boost immunity.

Vitamin E (tocopherol) is an antioxidant and is added to cosmetics for its ability to preserve oils. Topically, it can help minimize scarring and helps protect the skin against free radical damage.

Walnut (*Juglans nigra*, *J. regia*) is a member of the Juglandaceae (Walnut) Family. The leaves, inner bark, and outer rind of the unripe nut are used for their alterative, anti-inflammatory, antiseptic, and astringent properties. Walnut is used topically in salves to treat athlete's foot, eczema, fungal infection, herpes, impetigo, and ringworm. The hulls are used in shampoos and conditioners as a colorant to darken hair. The hulls are also used as a coloring agent for eyebrows and as an eye shadow; it is sometimes combined with tragacanth gum.

Watercress herb (*Nasturtium officinale*) is a member of the Brassicaceae (Cruciferous) Family. Watercress is a metabolic stimulant and highly nutritive; it should be eaten often. As a hair tonic, it encourages thick growth. The juice is applied to skin to clear acne, blemishes, eczema, and freckles. Applied as a facial mask, watercress leaves the skin smooth.

Watermelon (*Citrullus lanatus*, *C. vulgaris*) is a member of the Cucurbitaceae (Gourd) Family. Watermelon is considered a rejuvenating blood tonic and very alkalinizing. It is also antibacterial, antioxidant, diuretic, and laxative.

shampoos, hair dyes, conditioners, lotions, creams, and bubble baths.

- Esters are the result of mixing fatty alcohol with acids to act as stabilizers. Cetyl, cetearyl, stearic acid, and stearyl alcohols are all examples, and they serve as emulsifiers. The first word of an ester's name will end in "yl" and the second word will end in "ate." Some examples are glyceryl stearate, isopropyl palmitate, and tocopheryl linoleate. When a word ends in "yl," it is a fatty alcohol. An ending of "ate" indicates a fatty acid. There are exceptions, such as the sunscreen ingredient octyl methoxycinnamate.
- Fatty acids are produced in the body to form a moisturizing, gluelike compound that holds cells together and forms a protective barrier against the elements. Fatty acids are also used in cosmetics at amounts from 2–8 percent. They help smooth skin roughness and restore the skin's protective barrier without clogging pores. Examples of these acids include amino acids, hyaluronic acid, and nucleic acids (DNA, RNA); they all can help attract moisture.
- Fatty alcohols include cetearyl alcohol, cetyl alcohol, and stearyl alcohol. They are used as skin-softening emulsifiers to keep water and oil from separating. Some alcohols are moisture attracting and include butylenes glycol, glycerol, propylene, and sorbitol. Some vitamin ingredients can also be alcohols, such as vitamin E (tocopherol), vitamin A (retinol), panthenol (B_5), and cholecalciferol (vitamin D).
- Formaldehyde is used in many skin, hair, and nail products. It can be recognized

by words that include "form," such as "Formalin" and "formalith." Formaldehyde can cause skin and scalp irritation and is often listed as preservative quaternium-15 or quaternium 8-14.

- "Gly" usually indicates a humectant (water-attracting) substance.
- Imidazolidinyl urea is a preservative that is often added to soaps and shampoos to bind with metallic ions so that they do not impede the cleansing activity of the product. Although it can release formaldehyde into the product, it is considered nontoxic and nonirritating when used in small quantities.
- Mineral oil and petroleum jelly are by-products of the petroleum industry (leftovers from when crude oil is turned into refined oil) and do not break down readily. They dissolve the skin's natural oil, act as magnets for dirt, and can clog pores and aggravate acne. They do not contain minerals, have no nutritional value, and are a cheap alternative to natural oils. Mineral oil has large molecules that prevent absorption, causing the oil to stay on the top of the skin. This blocks sebum and impairs the body's ability to receive real moisture. Mineral oil can impede the assimilation of fat-soluble vitamins (A, D, E, and K). It is not recommended. Can you believe that this has long been the basic ingredient for commercial baby oils?
- Parabens (including methylparaben, propylparaben, and butylparaben) are preservatives that mimic estrogens. Their presence in underarm deodorants have been linked to an increased risk of breast

Watermelon is a good source of beta-carotene, vitamin C, potassium, and silicon. Watermelon makes an ideal food during a cleanse. In some parts of South America, watermelon rind is applied to the temples and forehead to cool a headache. Watermelon pulp is used topically to treat heat rash and burns. As a facial, it is astringent and refreshing.

Wheat germ oil is rich in beta-carotene, vitamins D and E, and lecithin. It is naturally antioxidant and helps prevent scarring. As it is sticky and thick, it is best to dilute it with other lighter oils. It has a tendency to go rancid easily.

White oak bark (*Quercus alba*) is a member of the Fagaceae (Beech) Family. It is rich in tannins, which cause its action to be very astringent. It is also very anti-inflammatory and antiseptic. The tannins bind with protein in the tissues making them impermeable to bacterial invasion and infection while fortifying the strength of the tissues. White oak is used as a compress, poultice, or salve for contact dermatitis, eczema, insect bites, ringworm, sties, and wounds. The galls are used as a coloring agent to darken the hair.

Wintergreen (*Gaultheria procumbens*) is a member of the Ericaceae (Heath) Family. The leaves and essential oil are both used for their analgesic, antiseptic, aromatic, astringent, and stimulant properties. The essential oil is used in massage oils to treat cellulite; it is also used in salves and lotions to remedy muscle and joint soreness. It is also employed in soaps for its fresh, zesty scent. Wintergreen is used in toothpastes and mouthwashes to freshen the breath.

Witch hazel (*Hamamelis virginiana*) is a member of the Hamamelidaceae (Witch Hazel) Family. The bark, twigs, and leaves are valued for their anti-inflammatory, antiseptic, astringent, cleansing, and styptic properties. Distilled witch hazel is commonly available at pharmacies. Witch hazel is used topically to treat acne, blemishes, bedsores, oily skin, insect bites, poison oak and ivy, and sunburn. Take care when using the distilled form close to your eyes and mucous membranes, as it contains rubbing alcohol, which can be an irritant. Witch hazel can also be used as a compress or salve to treat hemorrhoids and varicose veins. For treating dandruff and oily hair conditions, witch hazel is included in shampoos, conditioners, and hair rinses. Witch hazel is also applied as a deodorant and used as an aftershave.

Woodruff herb (*Asperula odorata*) is a member of the Rubiaceae (Madder) Family. The above-ground portions of the plant are used cosmetically for their anti-inflammatory properties. It is included in facial steams and as a bath herb. A poultice of the bruised leaves is used on boils and wounds. Its pleasant smell when dried is likened to freshly cut grass, vanilla, and honey, making it valuable in perfumes and soaps. It is also used in insect repellents.

Xanthan gum is a derivative of a fermented bacteria grown on corn sugar and used as a thickening agent in cosmetics.

Yarrow herb (*Achillea millefolium*), a member of the Asteraceae (Daisy) Family, is valued for its antifungal, anti-inflammatory, antiseptic, and astringent properties. The leaves and flowers are useful for oily skin in the form of facial steams, cleansers, and toners. It is used as a bath herb to treat rashes, wounds, and oily skin. In salves, yarrow is used to treat eczema. It is also used in aftershaves. Yarrow is a powerful styptic and a poultice of the fresh leaves will stop a wound from bleeding. Fresh yarrow can be rubbed on the skin to repel insects.

Yellow dock root (*Rumex crispus*) is a member of the Polygonaceae (Buckwheat) Family. This plant is valued for its alterative, antiseptic, astringent, and tonic properties. It aids the body's natural cleansing process. Rich in iron, it builds and purifies the blood. It is used internally to improve acne, boils, eczema, and psoriasis. It is employed in compresses, salves, and poultices for treating acne, eczema, hives, itchy skin, and ringworm.

Yerba maté (*Ilex paraguariensis*) is a member of the Aquifoliaceae (Holly) Family. The leaves are an alterative, antioxidant, antiscorbutic, aperient, astringent,

cancer. Parabens are also used in lipsticks, eye shadows, blushers, and foundations to increase their shelf life.

- Petroleum by-products include paraffin, mineral oil, petrolatum, isopropyl alcohol, carbomers, and microcrystalline wax. It has been estimated that up to 80 percent of all cosmetic ingredient formulations rely on petroleum and its by-products. Ingredients that might be derived in part from petroleum will contain the prefixes "butyl," "ethyl," "methyl," or "octyl." Petroleum-derived ingredients might also contain or end in one of the following: "PVP," "eth," or "ene."
- Ingredients that end in "ol" or "yl" are usually types of alcohol that serve as solvents and antiseptic agents.
- Phthalates are a group of synthetic chemicals, often labeled as DEP, DEHP, or DBP, that are used as chemical solvents and fragrance enhancers and to denature alcohol. They are sometimes referred to as plasticizers. In cosmetics they add luster to lotions, nail polishes, and hair sprays, and are also used to disperse fragrances. Most synthetic fragrances contain this ingredient. Phthalates can mimic estrogen and disrupt hormone functions.
- Preservatives are very difficult to avoid in most body care products. Without them, a product could readily be contaminated with bacteria, fungus, and/or mold. The preservatives ethylparaben, methylparaben, and propylparaben have been found to be mildly estrogenic. This group of preservatives, called parabens, are suspected carcinogens and can cause contact dermatitis; they

should be avoided. Quaternium-15, a commonly used cosmetic preservative, can cause allergic reactions. Hydantoin is a preservative that has been found to cause cancer in rats.

- The prefix "stear," as in stearic acid and stearyl alcohol, points to an ingredient that can either be plant (coconut or palm) or animal derived. It imparts a rich texture to cosmetic products. In some cases, this ingredient can be allergenic.
- Surfactants help to break up oils and create foam and thickness; they are used for cleansing the skin and body. Examples of surfactants are sodium lauryl sulfate and disodium lauryl sulfosuccinate. Milder surfactants include "ampho" (as in lauroamphocarboxyglycinate) or "betaine" (as in cocamidopropyl betaine). Sodium lauryl sulfate and sodium laureth sulfate are both found in many commercial products. When the suffix "eth" is present it indicates that the product has been modified in some way to reduce any irritating properties; thus, sodium laureth sulfate is considered milder and gentler than sodium lauryl sulfate. Many foam builders are synthetically produced, pollute our water supplies, and often are contaminated with nitrosamines that can cause cancer.
- Talc, also known as hydrous magnesium silicate, is used in powders. There has been a significant increase in ovarian cancers from those who have used powders containing talc in the genital region. Inhaling it can also cause respiratory distress. Talc should not be applied to babies or adults!

diaphoretic, diuretic, rejuvenative, stimulant, stomachic, and tonic. Maté cleanses the blood, stimulates the mind and respiratory and nervous systems, and decreases the appetite. It contains beta-carotene, vitamins B and C, calcium, iron, magnesium, manganese, potassium, silicon, sulfur, and tannins. The tannin content tends to bind with the caffeine in maté, thereby reducing the effects of both compounds. Most people who find caffeine impairs sleep will not experience this with maté. It is best to avoid consuming yerba maté with meals as the high tannin content can impair nutrient assimilation. Use cautiously if you suffer from anxiety, heart palpitations, and/or insomnia.

Ylang-ylang (*Cananga odorata*) is a member of the Annonaceae (Custard Apple) Family. The name means "flower of flowers," and the herb is used for its delightful fragrance. Ylang-ylang is used in skin products for oily and problem skin in the form of cleansers, soaps, toners, and moisturizers. It is also included in hair tonics, and the flowers can be rubbed directly on the hair if one is fortunate to live where the tree grows. This herb is sought after for its use in perfumery and is considered an aphrodisiac. Available as an absolute, it is euphoric, relaxes a nervous partner, and stimulates the senses. It has long been used to calm anger, anxiety, fear, frigidity, and improve self-esteem.

Yogurt contains lactic acid and encourages healthy intestinal flora when consumed. Of all the dairy products, it is the easiest to digest and the least allergenic. Use plain organic yogurt with active cultures. Topically, yogurt soothes the skin, is lightening, and improves large pores and oily, irritated, or blemished skin. It inhibits harmful bacteria that makes skin prone to blemishes.

Yucca root (*Yucca species*) is a member of the Agavaceae (Agave) Family. The roots are used for their anti-inflammatory properties. Yucca root contains saponins, which when mixed with water form a lather, making it an excellent biodegradable cleansing ingredient in shampoos, cleansers, and soaps. It is used for dandruff and hair loss, to soften hair, and to bring out highlights.

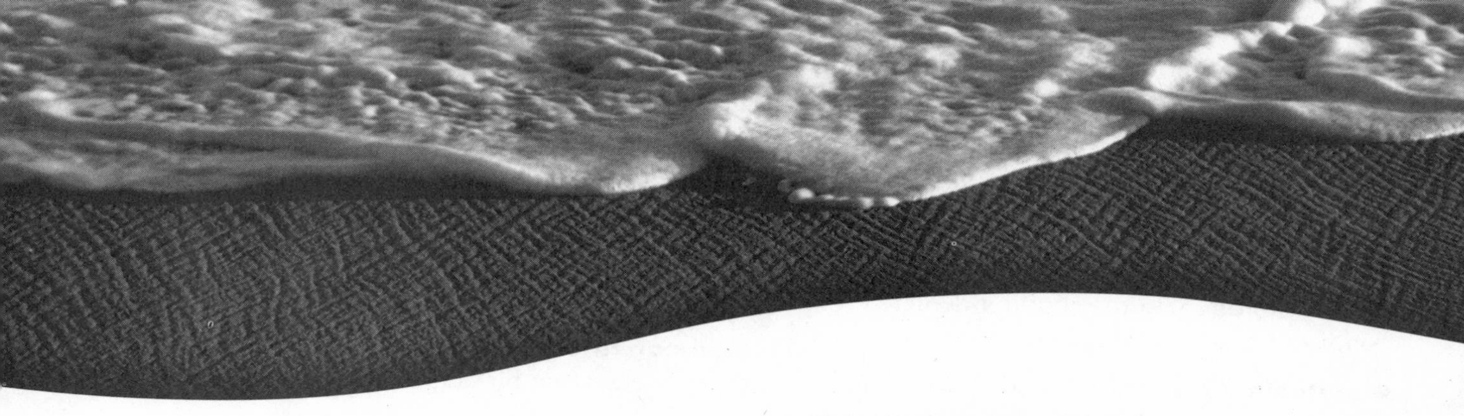

GLOSSARY

Adaptogens increase the body's resistance to stress and aid adaptation.

Alteratives modify or correct a condition. They increase blood flow to tissues and aid detoxification and excretion.

Analgesics relieve pain.

Anesthetics deaden sensation.

Anodynes are strong pain relievers that lessen nerve excitability.

Antifungals inhibit overgrowth of fungal organisms, such as *Candida*.

Anti-inflammatories soothe inflammation.

Antioxidants prevent free radical damage.

Antiseptics prevent bacterial growth, inhibit pathogens, and counter sepsis.

Antivirals inhibit viral replication.

Aphrodisiacs increase sexual desire and potency.

Aromatics are fragrant.

Astringents tighten, tone, dry secretions, and shrink blemishes. Many astringents contain tannins.

Bitters stimulate the flow of digestive, pituitary, liver, and duodenum secretions.

Calmatives are mildly sedating or tranquilizing.

Carminatives relieve gas and nausea.

Chi means "life force."

Demulcents soothe irritated tissues, especially mucous membranes in the throat.

Diaphoretics promote perspiration by relaxing the pores and increasing elimination through the skin.

Diuretics increase secretion and expulsion of urine by promoting activity of the kidneys and bladder.

Emollients are used externally to soothe, soften, and protect skin.

Hemostatics arrest bleeding and hemorrhaging.

Laxatives stimulate bowel action.

Mucilages are gelatinous substances that lubricate, soothe, and heal.

Nervines calm and nourish the nerves.

Nutritives are rich in nutrients and help build and tone the body.

Refrigerants are cooling, lower body temperature, and relieve thirst.

Rejuvenatives refresh and renew the body, mind, and spirit, and can slow down the aging process, counteract stress, and increase endurance.

Restoratives help to rebuild a depleted condition and restore normal body functions.

Rubefacients increase blood flow to the skin's surface and draw out deep impurities.

Sedatives slow down bodily actions and quiet the nerves.

Stimulants quicken various bodily actions, improve circulation, and warm the body.

Styptics stop bleeding by constricting blood vessels.

Tonics promote general health and well-being. They improve all organ systems and build energy, blood, and/or *chi*.

Vasoconstrictors narrow blood vessels, thereby elevating blood pressure.

Vasodilators expand blood vessels.

Vulneraries encourage wound healing by promoting cellular growth and repair.

BIBLIOGRAPHY

Arpel, Adrien, and Ronnie Sue Ebenstein. *Adrien Arpel's Three Week Crash Makeover/Shapeover Beauty Program*. New York: Rawson, 1977.

———. *How to Look Ten Years Younger*. New York: Rawson and Wade, 1980.

Avery, Alexandra. *Aromatherapy and You: A Guide to Natural Skin Care*. Kailua, HI: Blue Heron Hill, 1994.

Beckett, Sarah. *Herbs for Clearing the Skin*. Boulder, CO: Shambhala, 1980.

Begoun, Paula. *The Complete Beauty Bible: The Ultimate Guide to Smart Beauty*. Emmaus, PA: Rodale Press, 2004.

Benge, Sophie, and Luca Invernizzi. *Asian Secrets of Health, Beauty and Relaxation*. North Claredon, VT: Periplus, 2000.

Bragg, Paul C., and Patricia Bragg. *Your Health and Your Hair: Nature's Way to Beautiful Hair and Vibrant Health*. Santa Barbara, CA: Health Science, 1992.

Buchman, Diane Dincin. *The Complete Herbal Guide to Natural Health and Beauty*. New York: Doubleday, 1973.

Busch, Julia M. *Treat Your Face Like a Salad!* Coral Gables, FL: Anti-Aging Press, 1993.

Cameron, Myra. *Mother Nature's Guide to Vibrant Beauty and Health*. Englewood Cliffs, NJ: Prentice Hall, 1990.

Chang, Stephen. *The Crane Exercise: How to Rub Your Stomach Away*. Self-published, 1985.

Clark, Linda. *Linda Clark's Rejuvenation Programme: For Reversing the Ageing Process*. Wellingborough, England: Thorsons, 1980.

———. *Secrets of Health and Beauty: How to Make Yourself Over*. New York: Devin-Adair, 1969.

Clouatre, Dallas. *Getting Lean with Anti-Fat Nutrients*. San Francisco: Pax Publishing, 1993.

Cox, Janice. *Natural Beauty from the Garden: More Than 200 Do-It-Yourself Beauty Recipes and Garden Ideas*. New York: Henry Holt, 1999.

Cranshaw, Mary Ann. *The Natural Way to Super Beauty*. New York: D. McKay, 1974.

Dinsdale, Margaret. *Skin Deep: Natural Recipes for Healthy Skin and Hair*. Camden East, Ontario: Camden House, 1994.

Falconi, Dina. *Earthly Bodies and Heavenly Hair: Natural and Healthy Personal Care for Every Body*. Woodstock, NY: Ceres, 1998.

Frazier, Gregory, and Beverly Frazier. *The Bath Book*. San Francisco: Troubadour Press, 1973.

Freeman, Sally. *Everywoman's Guide to Ageless Natural Beauty*. Garden City, NY: GuildAmerica, 2000.

Genders, Roy. *Cosmetics from the Earth: A Guide to Natural Beauty*. New York: Alfred van der Marck, 1986.

Gittleman, Ann Louise, and Dina R. Nunziato. *Eat Fat, Lose Weight: How the Right Fats Can Make You Thin for Life*. Los Angeles: Keats, 1999.

Gladstar, Rosemary. *Herbs for Natural Beauty*. Pownal, VT: Storey Books, 1999.

Griscom, Chris. *The Ageless Body*. Galisteo, NM: Light Institute Press, 1992.

Grossbart, Ted A., and Carl Sherman. *Skin Deep: A Mind/Body Program for Healthy Skin*. Santa Fe, NM: Health Press, 1992.

Guyton, Anita. *Ageless Beauty the Natural Way*. London: Thorsons, 1993.

———. *The Natural Beauty Book: Cruelty Free Cosmetics to Make at Home*. London: Thorsons, 1992.

Hampton, Aubrey, and Susan Hussey. *The Take Charge Beauty Book: The Natural Guide to Beautiful Skin and Hair*. Tampa: Organica Press, 2000.

Irons, Diane. *911 Beauty Secrets*. Naperville, IL: Sourcebooks, 1999.

James, Kat. *The Truth about Beauty: Transform Your Looks and Your Life from the Inside Out*. Hillsboro, OR: Beyond Books, 2003.

Janssen, Mary Beth. *Naturally Healthy Hair: Herbal Treatments and Daily Care for Fabulous Hair*. Pownal, VT: Storey Books, 1999.

Johnson, Anne Akers. *The Body Book: Recipes for Natural Body Care*. Palo Alto, CA: Klutz, 2001.

Jones, Susan Smith. *Unleash the Power of Naturefoods: 50 Revitalizing Foods & Lifestyle Choices that Heal Your Body, Promote Radiant Health & Rejuvenate Your Life*. Salt Lake City, UT: Fine Living Books, 2005.

Kanner, Catherine. *The Book of the Bath*. New York: Fawcett Columbine, 1985.

Katzman, Shoshanna, Wendy Shankin-Cohen, and Melinda Marshall. *Feeling Light: The Holistic Solution to Permanent Weight Loss and Wellness*. New York: Avon, 1997.

Kellar, Casey. *The Natural Beauty and Bath Book: Nature's Luxurious Recipes for Body and Skin Care*. Asheville, NC: Lark Books, 1997.

Keller, Erich. *Aromatherapy Handbook for Beauty, Hair, and Skin Care*. Rochester, VT: Healing Arts, 1992.

Keuneke, Robin. *Total Breast Health: The Power Food Solution for Protection and Wellness*. New York: Kensington, 1998.

Keville, Kathi, and Mindy Green. *Aromatherapy: A Complete Guide to the Healing Art*. Freedom, CA: Crossing Press, 1995.

Lee, Helen. *The Tao of Beauty: Chinese Herbal Secrets to Feeling Good and Looking Great*. New York: Broadway, 1999.

Leigh, Michelle Dominique. *The Japanese Way of Beauty: Natural Beauty and Health Secrets*. New York: Carol Group, 1992.

Mars, Brigitte. *Herbal Pharmacy* (CD-ROM). Boulder, CO: Hale Enterprises, 1997.

McFarland, Judy Lindberg, and Laura McFarland Luczak. *Aging Without Growing Old*. Palos Verde, CA: Western Front, 1997.

Monte, Tom. *Staying Young: How to Prevent, Slow, or Reverse More Than 60 Signs of Aging*. Emmaus, PA: Rodale, 1994.

Moss, Susan. *Keep Your Breasts! Preventing Breast Cancer the Natural Way.* Los Angeles: Source Publications, 1994.

Perricone, Nicholas. *The Perricone Promise: Look Younger, Live Longer in Three Easy Steps*. New York: Warner, 2003.

Perry, Rachel. *Reverse the Aging Process of Your Face: A Simple Technique that Works*. Canoga Park, CA: Rachel Perry, Inc., 1979.

Prevention Magazine Health Books. *Age Erasers for Women: Actions You Can Take Right Now to Look Younger and Feel Great*. Emmaus, PA: Rodale Press, 1994.

Rees, Sian. *Natural Home Spa: Recreate the Luxurious Beauty Treatments of a Professional Spa in Your Own Home*. New York: Sterling, 1999.

Rose, Jeanne. *The Herbal Body Book*. New York: Berkley, 1982.

Schauss, Alexander, and Carolyn Costin. *Anorexia and Bulimia: A Nutritional Approach to the Deadly Eating Disorders*. New Canaan, CT: Keats, 1997.

Schrader, Constance. *No More Wrinkles: And 500 Other Foolproof Tips for Younger, Healthier Skin*. New York: New American Library, 1984.

Shaukat, Sidra. *Skin and Body Care: The Natural, Cruelty-Free Way to Beauty.* Rockport, MA: Element Books, 1992.

Singer, Sydney Ross, and Soma Grismaijer. *Dressed to Kill: The Link Between Breast Cancer and Bras*. Garden City Park, NY: Avery, 1995.

Somer, Elizabeth. *Age-Proof Your Body: Your Complete Guide to Lifelong Vitality.* New York: W. Morrow, 1998.

Tisserand, Maggie. *Essence of Love: Fragrance, Aphrodisiacs, and Aromatherapy for Lovers*. San Francisco: HarperCollins, 1993.

Tourles, Stephanie L. *The Herbal Body Book: A Natural Approach to Healthier Hair, Skin, and Nails*. Pownal, VT: Storey Books, 1994.

———. *Natural Foot Care: Herbal Treatments, Massage, and Exercises for Healthy Feet*. Pownal, VT: Storey Books, 1998.

Wesley-Hosford, Zia. *The Beautiful Body Book: A Lifetime Guide for Healthy, Younger-Looking Skin*. New York: Bantam Books, 1989.

———. *Face Value: Skin Care for Women Over 35*. San Francisco: Bantam Books, 1986.

Wesley-Hosford, Zia, and Mary Earle Chase. *Fifty and Fabulous: Zia's Definitive Guide to Anti-Aging, Naturally*. Rocklin, CA: Prima, 1995.

Wilson, Roberta. *A Complete Guide to Understanding and Using Aromatherapy for Vibrant Health & Beauty*. Garden City Park, NY: Avery, 1995.

Woodhall, Trinny, Susannah Constantine, and Robin Matthews. *What You Wear Can Change Your Life*. New York: Riverhead Books, 2005.

Yamaguchi, Billy. *Billy Yamaguchi Feng Shui Beauty*. Naperville, IL: Sourcebooks, 2004.

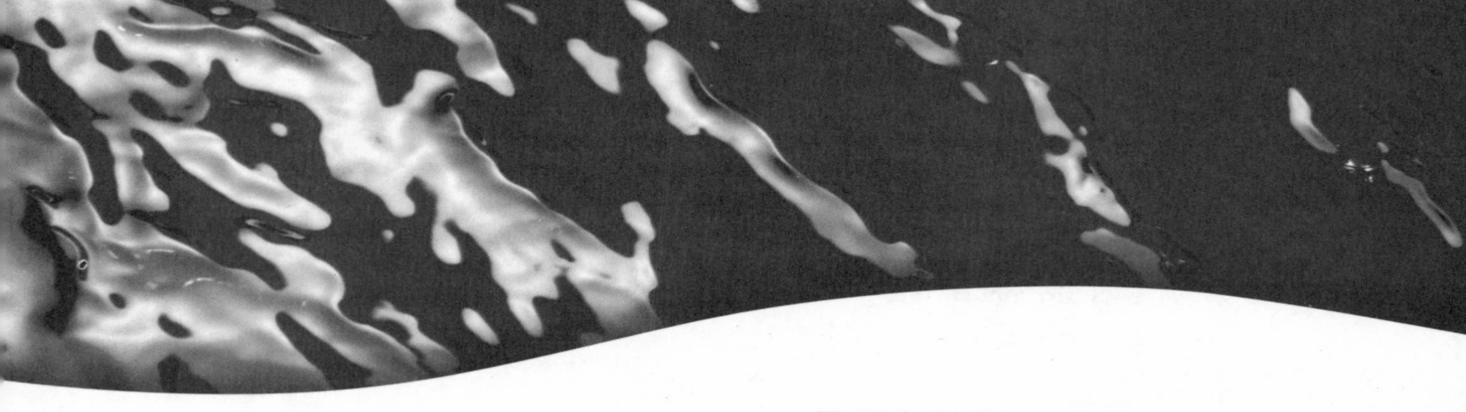

RESOURCES

Mail Order Suppliers

Many of the products listed in this book can be found in natural food and herbal stores; however, listed here are a few additional resources.

Age in Reverse

PO Box 1667
Newport Beach, CA 92663

800-443-3917

www.ageeasy.com

Slant boards and yoga tools.

American Herbalists Guild

141 Nob Hill Road
Cheshire, CT 06410

203-272-6731

www.americanherbalistsguild.com

Offers a directory of members of peer-reviewed herbal practitioners.

Aubrey Organics

4419 North Manhattan Avenue
Tampa, FL 33614

800-282-7394

www.aubrey-organics.com

Excellent natural products for skin and hair care.

Ball Beauty Supply

416 North Fairfax Avenue
Los Angeles, CA 90036

323-655-2330

www.ballbeauty.com

Sells Frownies, a wonderful beauty paste on tape that helps eliminate wrinkles.

Beauty Full You

1112 Montana #313
Santa Monica, CA 90403

310-571-3272

www.BeautyFullYou.com

One-stop shopping for the best beauty supplies, books, videos, and products. Hosted by supermodel Rainbeau Mars.

Colorganics, Inc.

PO Box 170507
San Francisco, CA 94117

877-524-4367

www.colorganics.net

Hemp-beeswax lipsticks.

Dr. Bronner's Magic Soaps

PO Box 28
Escondido, CA 92033

877-786-3649 or 760-743-2211

www.drbronner.com

Excellent peppermint and hemp-based soaps.

Dr. Hauschka Skin Care, Inc.

59 North Street
Hatfield, MA 01038

800-247-9907 or 413-247-9907

www.drhauschka.com

Quality botanically based cosmetics and body care products.

Essential Living Foods, Inc.

12304 Santa Monica Blvd., #218
Los Angeles, CA 90025

310-571-3272

www.essentiallivingfoods.com

The source for raw cacao, coconut oil, lycii berries, and the very best superfoods ever.

Frontier Herbs

PO Box 299
Norway, IA 52318

800-669-3275

www.frontiercoop.com

Mail-order herbs and herbal supplies.

Gaia Herbs

108 Island Ford Road
Brevard, NC 28712

888-917-8269 or 828-884-4242

www.gaiaherbs.com

Excellent herbal liquid extracts and Phyto-Caps, including Skin and Nail Support and many other herbal supplements.

Herb Pharm

PO Box 116
Williams, OR 97544

800-348-4372 or 541-846-6262

www.herb-pharm.com

My favorite company for herbal tinctures.

Horizon Herbs

PO Box 69
Williams, OR 97544-0069

541-846-6704

www.horizonherbs.com

A great source for herb seeds.

Little Moon Essentials

PO Box 771893
Steamboat Springs, CO 80477

888-273-0683

www.LittleMoonEssentials.com

Excellent aromatherapy bath, health, and body care products.

MegaFood

PO Box 325
Derry, NH 03038

800-848-2542

www.megafood.com

Makers of superior food-based vitamins.

Mountain Rose Herbs

PO Box 50220
Eugene, OR 97405

800-879-3337 or 541-741-7307

www.mountainroseherbs.com

Beeswax, bottles, misters, herbs, and essential oils.

National Association for Holistic Aromatherapy

3327 West Indian Trail Road
PMB 144
Spokane, WA 99208

888-275-6242 or 509-325-3419

www.naha.org

Where to learn about the practice of aromatherapy and aromatherapy products and practitioners.

Nature's First Law

PO Box 900202
San Diego, CA 92190

800-205-2350 or 619-596-7979

www.rawfood.com

Food, supplies, and books on a raw food diet.

Now and Zen

PO Box 110
Boulder, CO 80306

800-779-6383

www.now-zen.com

Alarm clocks that awaken you peacefully and other cosmic tools.

Original Swiss Aromatics

PO Box 6842
San Rafael, CA 94903

415-459-3998

www.originalswissaromatics.com

Purveyors of excellent essential oils.

Pangea Organics

6880 Winchester Circle, South Bay
Boulder, CO 80301

877-679-5854 or 303-413-8493

www.pangeaorganics.com

This company has a strong environmental commitment and makes superb body care products, some of which I formulated.

StarWest Botanicals

11253 Trade Center Drive
Rancho Cordova, CA 95742

800-800-4372 or 916-853-9354

www.starwest-botanicals.com

Mail-order herbs and herb supplies.

Vedic Harmonics Essential Oils

4926 Buchanan Place
Sarasota, FL 34231

941-929-0999

www.ayurvedichealers.com

I wholeheartedly support the quality of this line of essential oils and the environmental consciousness of the company.

Weleda

PO Box 675
Palisades, NY 10964

800-241-1030

www.usa.weleda.com

Sells botanical body care products.

Useful Web Sites

The Campaign for Safe Cosmetics

www.safecosmetics.org

Advocates for chemical-free cosmetics.

Health and Beauty America

www.hbaexpo.com

Sponsors beauty expos and conferences.

Informed Beauty

www.informedbeauty.com

Excellent articles on beauty from within.

The Trichological Society

www.hairscientists.org

Everything you might want to know about hair.

Other Publications by Brigitte Mars

Addiction-Free Naturally: Liberating Yourself from Sugar, Caffeine, Food Addictions, Tobacco, Alcohol, and Prescription Drugs. Rochester, VT: Healing Arts Press, 2001.

Dandelion Medicine: Remedies and Recipes to Detoxify, Nourish, Stimulate. North Adams, MA: Storey Publishing, 1999. Out of print; available in Chinese.

Elder: The Amazing Healing Benefits of Elder, the Premier Herbal Remedy for Colds and Flu. New Canaan, CT: Keats Publishing, Inc., 1997.

Healing Herbal Teas: A Complete Guide to Making Delicious, Healthful Beverages. North Bergen, NJ: Basic Health Publications, 2005.

HempNut Cookbook: Tasty, Omega-rich Meals from Hempseed. Coauthored with Richard Rose and edited by Christina Pirello. Summertown, TN: Book Publishing Company, 2004.

Herbs for Healthy Skin, Hair & Nails: Banish Eczema, Acne and Psoriasis with Healing Herbs that Cleanse the Body Inside and Out. New Canaan, CT: Keats Publishing, 1998.

Natural First Aid: Herbal Treatments for Ailments & Injuries, Emergency Preparedness, Wilderness Safety. North Adams, MA: Storey Publishing, 1999. Spanish version available.

Rawsome!: Maximizing Health, Energy, and Culinary Delight with the Raw Foods Diet. North Bergen, NJ: Basic Health Publications, 2004.

Sex, Love & Health: A Self-Help Health Guide to Love & Sex. North Bergen, NJ: Basic Health Publications, 2002.

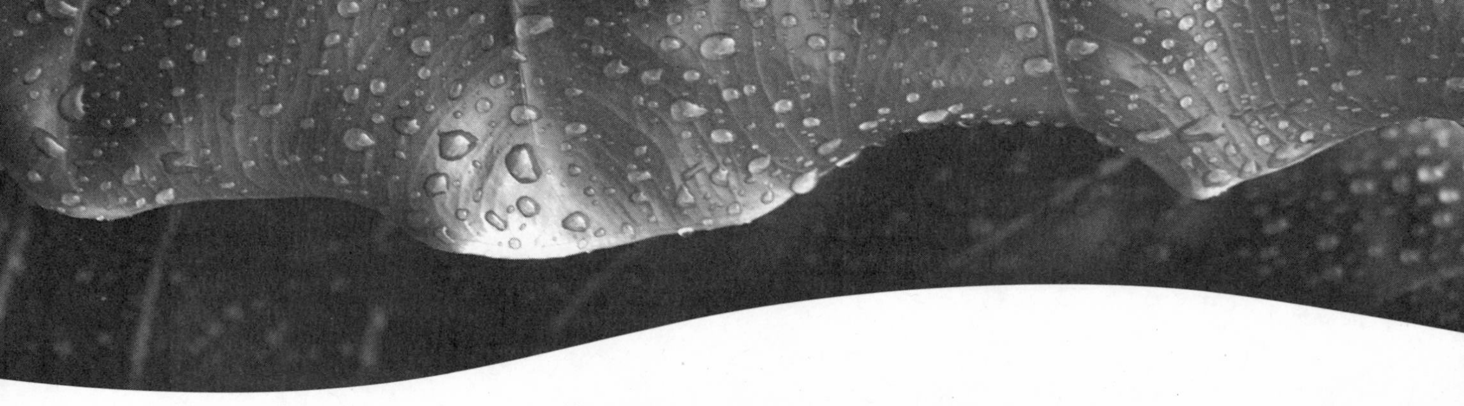

ABOUT THE AUTHOR

Brigitte Mars is an herbalist from Boulder, Colorado, with over thirty-five years of experience in natural medicine and is a founding and professional member of the American Herbalist Guild. She is the author of *Addiction-Free Naturally; Sex, Love and Health; Rawsome!;* and *Healing Herbal Teas,* and a co-author of *The HempNut Cookbook.* Brigitte has also written for magazines such as *Yoga Journal, Mothering, Natural Health,* and *Delicious Living.*

Brigitte teaches at Naropa University, Esalen Institute, Kripalu, Boulder College of Massage, and many other locations. She has a nutritional and herbal private practice and a local weekly radio show called *Naturally.*

Brigitte is the mother of Sunflower Sparkle Mars, with whom she leads Herb Camp for Kids, and Rainbeau Harmony Mars, who is an actress, model, and yogini living in Santa Monica (www.rainbeaumars.com). She has been happily married for over thirty years to human design analyst Tom Pfeiffer, with whom she teaches raw food workshops. They have two grandchildren.

For booking public speaking, herb walks, raw food classes, formulations, and health consultations, contact Brigitte at:

Brigitte@indra.com

303-442-4967

www.brigittemars.com

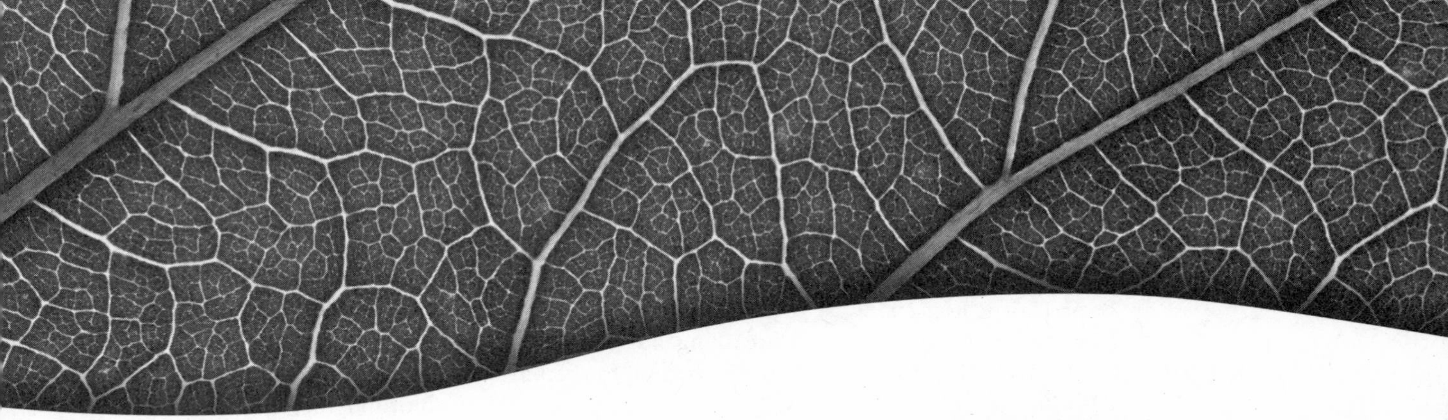

INDEX